Education in Oral and Maxillofacial Surgery: an Evolving Paradigm

Editors

LESLIE R. HALPERN
ERIC R. CARLSON

ORAL AND MAXILLOFACIAL SURGERY CLINICS OF NORTH AMERICA

www.oralmaxsurgery.theclinics.com

Consulting Editor
RUI P. FERNANDES

November 2022 • Volume 34 • Number 4

ELSEVIER

1600 John F. Kennedy Boulevard • Suite 1800 • Philadelphia, Pennsylvania, 19103-2899

http://www.oralmaxsurgery.theclinics.com

**ORAL AND MAXILLOFACIAL SURGERY CLINICS OF NORTH AMERICA Volume 34, Number 4
November 2022 ISSN 1042-3699, ISBN-13: 978-0-323-98705-9**

Editor: John Vassallo; j.vassallo@elsevier.com
Developmental Editor: Jessica Nicole B. Cañaberal

Oral and Maxillofacial Surgery Clinics of North America (ISSN 1042-3699) is published quarterly by Elsevier Inc., 360 Park Avenue South, New York, NY 10010-1710. Months of issue are February, May, August, and November. Business and Editorial Offices: 1600 John F. Kennedy Blvd., Suite 1800, Philadelphia, PA 19103-2899. Periodicals postage paid at New York, NY and additional mailing offices. Subscription prices are $405.00 per year for US individuals, $961.00 per year for US institutions, $100.00 per year for US students/residents, $478.00 per year for Canadian individuals, $990.00 per year for Canadian institutions, $100.00 per year for Canadian students/residents, $530.00 per year for international individuals, $990.00 per year for international institutions and $235.00 per year for international students/residents. To receive student/resident rate, orders must be accompanied by name or affiliated institution, date of term, and the *signature* of program/residency coordinator on institution letterhead. Orders will be billed at individual rate until proof of status is received. Foreign air speed delivery is included in all *Clinics* subscription prices. All prices are subject to change without notice. **POSTMASTER:** Send address changes to *Oral and Maxillofacial Surgery Clinics of North America,* Elsevier Periodicals **Customer Service, 11830 Westline Industrial Drive, St. Louis, MO 63146. Tel: 1-800-654-2452 (U.S. and Canada); 314-447-8871 (outside U.S. and Canada). Fax: 314-447-8029. E-mail: journalscustomerservice-usa@elsevier.com (for print support); journalsonlinesupport-usa@elsevier.com (for online support).**

Reprints. For copies of 100 or more, of articles in this publication, please contact the Commercial Reprints Department, Elsevier Inc., 360 Park Avenue South, New York, NY 10010-1710. Tel.: 212-633-3874; Fax: 212-633-3820; Email: reprints@elsevier.com.

Oral and Maxillofacial Surgery Clinics of North America is covered in *MEDLINE/PubMed (Index Medicus), Science Citation Index Expanded (SciSearch®), Journal Citation Reports/Science Edition,* and *Current Contents®/Clinical Medicine.*

Contributors

CONSULTING EDITOR

RUI P. FERNANDES, MD, DMD, FACS, FRCS(Ed)
Clinical Professor and Chief, Division of Head and Neck Surgery, Program Director, Head and Neck Oncologic Surgery and Microvascular Reconstruction Fellowship, Departments of Oral and Maxillofacial Surgery, Neurosurgery, and Orthopaedic Surgery and Rehabilitation, University of Florida Health Science Center, University of Florida College of Medicine, Jacksonville, Florida

EDITORS

LESLIE R. HALPERN, DDS, MD, PhD, MPH, FACS, FICD
Professor, Section Chief, Program Director, OMFS Residency, New York Medical College/Metropolitan Hospital of NYCHHC, New York, New York; Professor, Section Head, Oral and Maxillofacial Surgery, University of Utah, School of Dentistry, Salt Lake City, Utah

ERIC R. CARLSON, DMD, MD, EdM, FACS
Professor, Kelly L. Krahwinkel Endowed Chairman, Department of Oral and Maxillofacial Surgery, University of Tennessee Graduate School of Medicine Knoxville, Tennessee

AUTHORS

ROBERT BRUCE DONOFF, DMD, MD, FACD, FACS
Walter Guralnick Distinguished Professor of Oral and Maxillofacial Surgery, Harvard University Distinguished Service Professor

LEON A. ASSAEL, DMD
Adjunct Clinical Professor, Department of Restorative and Preventive Dentistry, University of California, San Francisco, San Francisco, California; Emeritus Dean and Professor of Oral and Maxillofacial Surgery, University of Minnesota, Minneapolis, Minnesota; Retired Professor and Chair, Oral and Maxillofacial Surgery, Oregon Health & Science University, Portland, Oregon

ERIC R. CARLSON, DMD, MD, EdM, FACS
Professor, Kelly L. Krahwinkel Endowed Chairman, Department of Oral and Maxillofacial Surgery, University of Tennessee Graduate School of Medicine Knoxville, Tennessee

LARRY L. CUNNINGHAM, JR., DDS, MD, FACS
Professor and Chair, Department of Oral and Maxillofacial Surgery, Associate Dean of Hospital Affairs, University of Pittsburgh School of Dental Medicine, Pittsburgh, Pennsylvania

ERIC J. DIERKS, MD, DMD, FACS, FACD, FRCS(Ed)
Affiliate Professor, Department of Oral and Maxillofacial Surgery, Oregon Health & Science University, Head and Neck Surgical Associates, Portland, Oregon

STEPHANIE J. DREW, DMD, FACS
Associate Professor, Department of Surgery, Division of Oral and Maxillofacial Surgery, Emory University, Atlanta, Georgia

JULIE GLOWACKI, PhD
Professor of Orthopedic Surgery and of Oral and Maxillofacial Surgery Emerita, Department of Orthopedic Surgery, Brigham and Women's Hospital, Harvard Medical School, Harvard School of Dental Medicine, Boston, Massachusetts

ROBERT HALE, DDS
COL (Ret), US Army, Woodland Hills, California

LESLIE R. HALPERN, DDS, MD, PhD, MPH, FACS, FICD
Professor, Section Chief, Program Director, OMFS Residency, New York Medical College/Metropolitan Hospital of NYCHHC, New York, New York; Professor, Section Head, Oral and Maxillofacial Surgery, University of Utah, School of Dentistry, Salt Lake City, Utah

JACK A. HARRIS, DMD
Harvard School of Dental Medicine, Boston, Massachusetts

CATHERINE HORAN, PhD
Retired Consultant, Accreditation for the Commission on Dental Accreditation

JAMES R. HUPP, DMD, MD, JD, MBA
Senior Associate Dean for Policy and Compliance, Interim Chief Health Officer, Elson S. Floyd College of Medicine, Washington State University, Spokane, Washington

YISI D. JI, MD, DMD
Harvard Medical School, Boston, Massachusetts

LEONARD B. KABAN, DMD, MD, FACS
Walter C. Guralnick Distinguished Professor and Chief Emeritus, Department of Oral and Maxillofacial Surgery, Massachusetts General Hospital, Harvard School of Dental Medicine, Boston, Massachusetts

DEEPAK G. KRISHNAN, DDS
Associate Professor of Surgery, Chief of Oral and Maxillofacial Surgery, University of Cincinnati, Cincinnati, Ohio

EILEEN MCGOWAN, EdD
Former Director, Specialized Studies Program, Harvard Graduate School of Education, Cambridge, Massachusetts

VINCENT J. PERCIACCANTE, DDS, FACS
Adjunct Associate Professor of Surgery, Division of Oral and Maxillofacial Surgery, Emory University School of Medicine, Atlanta, Georgia; Private Practice, South Oral and Maxillofacial Surgery, Peachtree City, Georgia

DAVID H. PERROTT, DDS, MD, MBA, FACS
Former Senior Vice President and Chief Medical Officer, California Hospital Association, Phoenix, Arizona

STEVEN ROSER, MD, DMD, FACS, FRCSEd
Delos Hill Chair and Professor of Surgery, Residency Program Director, Division of Oral and Maxillofacial Surgery, Department of Surgery, Emory University School of Medicine, Chief of Oral and Maxillofacial Surgery, Grady Memorial Hospital, Atlanta, Georgia

SRUTHI SATISHCHANDRAN, DMD
Resident-in-Training, Oral and Maxillofacial Surgery, Emory University School of Medicine, Atlanta, Georgia

JONATHAN W. SHUM, MD, DDS, FACS, FRCD(D)
Associate Professor, Fellowship Director, Founder of Oral, Head and Neck Oncologic and Reconstructive Surgery Fellowship, Department of Oral and Maxillofacial Surgery, The University of Texas Health Science Center at Houston, Houston, Texas

R. JOHN TANNYHILL III, DDS, MD, FACS
Oral and Maxillofacial Surgery Residency Program Director and Education Director, Massachusetts General Hospital, Assistant Professor, Harvard School of Dental Medicine, Boston, Massachusetts

Contents

> This article highlights the needs in dental education for more general medicine and scientific information. The author suggests that oral and maxillofacial surgeons could have an important role to play in this education beyond surgical procedures. The Educational Committee of AAOMS has made this point prepandemic, and it is more important now. As the patient population ages, this role assumes greater importance. Patients now have more chronic diseases and take more medicines, and the repertoire and scope of practice for dentists should be improved to care for the general health of patients. Our specialty should play a leadership role in the transformation of the profession.

> Here, we trace the history of oral and maxillofacial surgery (OMS) education from the mid-19th century to the present. We consider the effects of separation of dentistry and medicine, discovery of anesthesia, antisepsis, antibiotics, and wars on surgical progress and training. In the 19th century, apprenticeships with well-known surgeons were the norm. In the 20th century, training evolved from nonintegrated dental school and hospital experiences to 3- and then 4-year integrated hospital programs. After World War II individual oral surgeons pursued the MD degree after residency. The formal dual degree OMS paradigm began in the 1970s.

> The goal of graduate surgical education is to ensure that the graduate is competent to practice in his or her chosen specialty. Traditionally, surgical learning has been based on an apprenticeship model; that is, the long-term observation and assessment of the trainee over a prolonged period of time. Patient expectations, work hour restrictions, and expectations of increased faculty oversight have led to decreased resident autonomy and independence. Graduates completing surgical training with less surgical autonomy may have lower clinical competence, which may affect patient safety, patient outcomes, and career satisfaction. This will require the modification of current assessment and training methods.

and the American higher education environment. A changing workforce and practice model combined with today's technology revolution are being incorporated into OMS residency education.

Jonathan W. Shum and Eric J. Dierks

The pursuit of fellowship training stems from one's desire to master a focused area of surgery. Successful applicants tend to have published articles and participated in other scholarly activities. They commonly have a mentor within the subspecialty of their interest. Selection of the program is generally based on the breadth of experience available followed by faculty reputation and location. Advantages to the successful fellowship graduate include the experience and confidence to provide specialized and efficient care to patients. Enhancements to an academic department with a fellowship program include mentorship for residents and guidance toward fellowship, as well as an increased level of scholarly activity.

Eric R. Carlson and Eileen McGowan

Faculty development is a poorly understood and incompletely executed initiative in undergraduate and graduate medical and dental education programs. Despite significant change in the delivery of health care over the past several decades, the education of students and residents has followed a legacy path of business as usual. Some faculty have incorrectly assumed that content expertise transfers to teaching expertise. The insistence for robust faculty development programs on the part of accrediting and other professional organizations has created a call to action, but much work has yet to be done. It is therefore essential that leaders in these programs develop a sense of urgency to teach the teachers lest our students and residents will replicate outdated methods, unsystematically teach themselves, and fall victim to an educational system that is grossly inadequate. It is the purpose of this article to enhance undergraduate and graduate medical and dental education by offering viable change options, specifically targeted to improving historical trends by emphasizing the importance of growth mindsets, emotional intelligence, the creation of holding environments, and stimulating enthusiasm for lifelong learning as part of twenty-first century strategies for faculty development.

James R. Hupp and Leslie R. Halpern

Mentoring, coaching, role modeling, and teaching all represent strategies in which one or more individuals help develop another individual. Although there are some similarities among those providing the guidance to the recipient of the development efforts, important differences exist. This article defines and discusses the similarities and differences between these roles. It goes on to focus on how surgical residents can best be served by mentors, coaches, role models, and teachers in their journey to becoming practicing surgeons. Guidance on how to best serve in one of these roles is provided along with guidance on how a surgical resident can take advantage of this excellent form of career development.

The importance of active adult learning methods and critical thinking skills is appreciated in dental and OMFS residency training. Known barriers to research are finding time in the curriculum and funding needed for research experiences. These barriers have inspired many institutions to design programs to provide research opportunities, but they can be expensive and of minimal interest to those not planning academic careers. During OMFS residency training, the primary emphasis is on mastery of all aspects of surgical care. Strong partnerships between PhD researchers and OMFS clinical investigators, formed to advance the field, can also have an impact on trainees' involvement in research and their understanding of rigorous evidence-based principles of clinical care.

Artificial intelligence has become ubiquitous with modern technology. Digital transformations are occurring in every field including medicine, surgery, and education. Computers and computer programs are getting sophisticated to form neural networks globally. These algorithms allow for sophisticated and complex pattern recognitions and make accurate predictions. This allows for both accurate diagnosis and prognostication in medicine and opens opportunities for medical and surgical education. Oral and Maxillofacial surgeons and OMS education like all of the surgery are adapting well to the world of AI, incorporating machine learning into simulation, and attaching sensors to master surgeons to understand motion economy.

Achieving technical excellence in surgery can happen at any point of a surgical career. The accumulation of wisdom brought by the aging surgeon's decades of experience, however, can only come with time and practice. With the accumulated life and professional experience obtained, aging surgeons can still contribute a valuable perspective/point of view to young trainees and colleagues. This article reviews the current literature of the aging surgeon and suggests strategies for how aging surgeons can use their expertise in an innovative fashion to train and develop the future legacy of the specialty.

ORAL AND MAXILLOFACIAL SURGERY CLINICS OF NORTH AMERICA

SERIES OF RELATED INTEREST

Atlas of the Oral and Maxillofacial Surgery Clinics
www.oralmaxsurgeryatlas.theclinics.com

Dental Clinics
www.dental.theclinics.com

ORAL AND MAXILLOFACIAL SURGERY
CLINICS OF NORTH AMERICA

FORTHCOMING ISSUES

February 2023
Global Perspectives in Contemporary
Orthognathic Surgery
Mike Yiu Yan Leung, Editor

May 2023
Diagnosis and Management of Oral Mucosal
Lesions
Paul C Edwards and Donald Cohen, Editors

August 2023
Imaging of the Common Oral Cavity,
Sinonasal, and Skull Base Pathology
Dinesh Rao, Editor

RECENT ISSUES

August 2022
Craniosynostosis: Current Perspectives
Srinivas M Susarla, Editor

May 2022
Management of Melanoma of the Head and
Neck
Al Haitham Al Shetawi, Editor

February 2022
Clinical Pharmacology for the Oral and
Maxillofacial Surgeon
Harry Dym, Editor

SERIES OF RELATED INTEREST

Atlas of the Oral and Maxillofacial Surgery Clinics
www.oralmaxsurgeryatlas.theclinics.com

Dental Clinics
www.dental.theclinics.com

Dedication

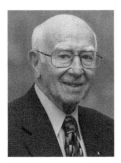

Daniel Laskin, DDS (September 3, 1924–December 8, 2021)

We dedicate this issue of the *Oral and Maxillofacial Surgery Clinics of North America* to the memory of Dr Daniel Laskin. Dr Laskin was internationally renowned in the specialty of Oral and Maxillofacial Surgery. He was the consummate educator, who taught those around him to be dedicated to our profession and to the patients for whom we care. Dr Laskin believed that each of us should be committed to serving as a mentor to those we teach while being committed to lifelong learning within our specialty. He was the quintessential researcher, and he thought critically about global issues in health care. Dr Laskin served numerous academic centers, including the University of Illinois at Chicago and the Virginia Commonwealth University, where he was active until the time of his passing on December 8, 2021. Dr Laskin was perhaps best known for having served as the Editor-in-Chief of the *Journal of Oral and Maxillofacial Surgery* from 1972 to 2002, during which time he provided oversight of the research and publications that have served to shape the clinical practice of Oral and Maxillofacial Surgery. He also served as editor of *AAOMS Today*, and he received numerous honors and accolades, including the 2018 Distinguished Dental Editor Award from the American Dental Association's Council on Communications and the American Association of Dental Editors

and Journalists. Dr Laskin was President of the American Association of Oral and Maxillofacial Surgeons from 1976 to 1977, and President of the International Association of Oral and Maxillofacial Surgeons from 1983 to 1986.

Our specialty has lost a beloved member of its family, but we are mindful of the legacy he crafted in education. Dr Daniel Laskin will be remembered fondly and missed greatly by all. To this end, we proudly dedicate this issue to the memory of Dr Daniel Laskin.

Leslie R. Halpern, DDS, MD, PhD, MPH, FACS, FICD
New York Medical College/Metropolitan Hospital of NYCHHC of New York/
1901 First Avenue, NYC, NY 10029, USA

Eric R. Carlson, DMD, MD, EdM, FACS
Department of Oral and Maxillofacial Surgery
University of Tennessee Graduate School of Medicine
Knoxville, TN 37920, USA

E-mail addresses:
leslie.halpern@hsc.utah.edu (L.R. Halpern)
Ecarlson@utmck.edu (E.R. Carlson)

Oral Maxillofacial Surg Clin N Am 34 (2022) xi
https://doi.org/10.1016/j.coms.2022.07.002
1042-3699/22/© 2022 Published by Elsevier Inc.

Preface

Education in Oral and Maxillofacial Surgery: An Evolving Paradigm

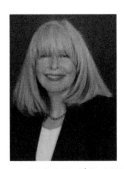
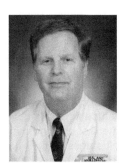

Leslie R. Halpern, DDS, MD, PhD, MPH, FACS, FICD   Eric R. Carlson, DMD, MD, EdM, FACS

Editors

Undergraduate and graduate medical and dental education has undergone a transformation since its dawn in the early twentieth century, transitioning from a proprietary apprenticeship model toward a more robust framework based on basic science, research, and hands-on patient care in academic health center arenas. This traditional Halsteadian model laid the foundation for a formal approach to education that forms the algorithms that educators now follow with an emphasis on evidence-based best practices in patient care. There continues to be the need, however, to develop new curricula and new methods of teaching that will meet the challenges of oral and maxillofacial surgery education in the twenty-first century. The benchmark criteria for accreditation standards of the Commission on Dental Accreditation, the attainment of educational competencies for board certification by the American Board of Oral and Maxillofacial Surgery, changes in technology, legitimate programs in faculty development, and the dynamics of health policy will continue to influence the clinical and didactic training of our residents in our specialty. An in-depth understanding of all of these issues has the potential to create an effective construct in meeting the challenges of contemporary oral and maxillofacial surgery education while creating bona fide learning environments. Oral and maxillofacial surgery educators must therefore re-craft curricular standards that are grounded in traditional standards of care, the dynamics of evidence-based outcomes, evolving technology, and new educational models that will enhance life-long learning in clinical practice. Effectively educating competent surgeons requires innovative and high-quality educational methods, with the recognition that the surgical classroom is subject to transformational change based on an understanding of the contemporary learner and learning styles. Coregulated learning permits faculty and residents to form collaborative approaches to patient care that enhance the quality of supervised learning. Learning and teaching are bidirectional such that a dynamic exists of educating the educator. Interactive learning platforms convert superficial learning to deep learning. With the growth of technology, there has been an increase in use of simulation, including virtual reality, robotics, telemedicine, and artificial intelligence. These approaches allow the surgical learner to apply novel principles to gain information, including online surgical resources, videos, podcasts, and social media. Their use has shifted the learning of basic surgical skills to the laboratory, thereby augmenting the operating room experience of the acquisition of complex surgical skills. This approach provides surgical educators with a foundational framework of innovative techniques that promote resident and student learning, and faculty development programs reinforce the sustainability of these techniques. Finally, the creation of online curricula allows educators to overcome obstacles related to surgical education

Oral Maxillofacial Surg Clin N Am 34 (2022) xiii–xiv
https://doi.org/10.1016/j.coms.2022.07.001
1042-3699/22/© 2022 Published by Elsevier Inc.

with increased accessibility of learning material, ease in updating and editing content, personalized instruction, ease of distribution, calibration of surgical content, and learner accountability.

We are privileged to provide an issue of the *Oral and Maxillofacial Surgery Clinics of North America* focusing on an evolving paradigm of education of residents in our specialty. Our participation as surgical educators places us in a pivotal position to produce an insightful group of visionary educators in oral and maxillofacial surgery who are brought to the table to create a thought-provoking roadmap that will enhance strategies for the education of members of our specialty. A compelling argument is made for transformational change in the education of predoctoral students, residents, and the professional development of oral and maxillofacial surgery faculty at all stages of their career who are committed to providing the education of a new generation of surgeons. We wish to extend our thanks to John Vassallo, editor of *Oral and Maxillofacial Surgical Clinics of North America*, and Dr Rui Fernandes, Consulting Editor, for his support and encouragement of this project. We thank our current and former students, residents, and fellows, whom we have had the privilege of teaching. Our relationships embody the definition of academic oral and maxillofacial surgery, and we strive to continue to meet their expectations as surgeon educators.

Leslie R. Halpern, DDS, MD, PhD, MPH, FACS, FICD
New York Medical College/ Metropolitan Hospital of NYCHHC
1901 First Avenue
New York, NY 10029, USA

Eric R. Carlson, DMD, MD, EdM, FACS
Department of Oral and Maxillofacial Surgery
University of Tennessee Graduate School of Medicine
Knoxville, TN 37920, USA

E-mail addresses:
Halpernl@nychhc.org (L.R. Halpern)
Ecarlson@utmck.edu (E.R. Carlson)

Predoctoral Dental Education

The Changing Role and Growing Importance of Oral and Maxillofacial Surgery and Surgeon Teachers Innovation Versus Incumbency

Robert Bruce Donoff, DMD, MD

KEYWORDS

• Integration of medicine and science • Patient centered • Problem based • Simulation

KEY POINTS

• Oral and maxillofacial surgeons should assume more teaching of general medicine for dental students.
• Full-time faculty will improve dental education.
• CAree of the whole patient is critical.

INTRODUCTION

In 2016, I coauthored an article in these Clinics with Dr Sara Gordon on interprofessional education (IPE).[1] At that time, many believed that IPE could be the answer to broadening the education of dental students in areas of general patient care, pharmacology, and understanding of comorbid disease in dental patients. My thoughts were that too much of IPE was aligned with nursing, pharmacy, and not medicine, and dependence on multiple schedules was difficult. Now, I find myself charged with discussing predoctoral dental education because it applies to oral and maxillofacial surgery. The experience for predoctoral dental students varies from school to school but learning still deals with several major areas. These are general knowledge of the field, diagnosis of pathologic conditions, and surgical methods of treatment. Although some of my ideas work in the current COVID environment, clearly a return to normal is preferred. The more important issue is the quality

and impact of dental education on patient care and outcomes as dentists care for older patients with more chronic diseases and taking more medicines.[2] This is particularly relevant for oral and maxillofacial surgery because such procedures often provide great anxiety and general concern. Often such procedures require sedation or even general anesthesia, areas of potential teaching and learning of pulmonary and cardiovascular physiology. I believe that dental education must change if the profession is to function best in our health-care system. Baring greater integration with medicine in learning and practice,[3] in my opinion, faculty OMFSs have a potentially major role in righting the lack of basic science and medicine in the dental students' preparation in addition to providing the basics of learning for the diagnosis and management of head and neck pathologies, such as cysts and oral cancer. All dentists should be knowledgeable as to what conditions or suspicions should be referred to an OMFS. This will require a concerted effort of faculty in dental

Department of Oral and Maxillofacial Surgery, Harvard School of Dental Medicine, 188 Longwood Avenue, Boston, MA, USA
E-mail address: bruce_donoff@hsdm.harvard.edu

Oral Maxillofacial Surg Clin N Am 34 (2022) 489–493
https://doi.org/10.1016/j.coms.2022.03.010
1042-3699/22/© 2022 Elsevier Inc. All rights reserved.

schools, faculty in residency programs, and the support of leadership in dental schools. The scope and depth of dental education has changed so that procedures rule the curriculum. Testing methods support and promote this and the continued lack of a general practice year for all graduates eliminates an important place for learning about patient illness and its management.[4] At my institution, the attractiveness of oral surgery is enhanced by an integrated medical curriculum for part of the doctor of dental medicine (DMD) program and preparation for learning how to take a history, learn about the patient from the patient, and consideration of all the chronic conditions and medications that a patient may take and not only from a computer screen checklist. My proudest moments as Dean came during commencement, when degrees were awarded and the President of the University welcomed the graduates into a demanding branch of medicine.

Historical Aspects Teaching Medicine

The separation of dental and medical education, practice, and payment mechanisms are major problems in closing the division between oral health and overall health.[5] Progress has been steady but slow, probably because the focus has been more on changing the structures that hold the separation in place with less attention on the people in the system who create and uphold the structures and the overall culture. How students are educated and trained is critical.

What are the goals of having dental students and practitioners understand the impact of medical conditions on their treatments.[6] The goal is better patient care and outcomes. The population is aging and multimorbidity of chronic disease is a major issue. Watt and Serban state very directly the following. "Over the last 30 years, considerable efforts have been made to better integrate the training of oral health professionals within the wider healthcare educational system. However much, if not most, of dental professional undergraduate, postgraduate and continuing professional development courses still continue to be delivered in an isolated and compartmentalized fashion, separated from the mainstream training of other health professionals. This siloed approach to professional education needs to radically change if the future oral health workforce is going to be equipped with the knowledge, skills and competencies needed to provide high-quality and integrated care to the ever-increasing numbers of patients with multiple health conditions." Truly integrated models of education and training are needed, which include a significant focus on multimorbidity

(in terms of common social determinants, pathogenesis, treatment modalities, and impact), and the best ways of addressing and supporting the (oral) health needs of patients with multiple conditions. Greater emphasis needs to be placed on training oral health professionals to be active and core members of multidisciplinary health teams working in primary care, community, or hospital settings. Undergraduate and continuing professional development training also needs to equip oral health professionals with highly developed communication skills to enable them to communicate effectively with other health professionals, as well as with patients and their families living with complex health needs. It is also very important that core oral health input is included in the curriculum and assessment of medical, pharmacy, and nursing students to ensure that they are better informed and equipped to deal with oral health problems, and when appropriate to refer patients to oral health professionals.[7]

The oral surgeon teacher can have a major impact on student learning of medical management. One of the most obvious is related to anticoagulants. When I was "growing up," there were only 2 blood thinners, warfarin and coumadin; now, there are many more. Understanding the reasons for anticoagulation informs medical learning, and understanding the direct oral anticoagulants versus the vitamin K antagonists warfarin and the use of PT, partial prothromin time (PTT), and INR is a meaningful exercise for student learning of the biochemistry of health care. Most studies support the clinical decision not to alter DOACs for most dental extractions.[8,9]

Teaching about cardiovascular disease, stroke, and arrythmias can be done by the oral surgeon teacher prepared to do this in the curricular development. Similar teaching exercises can be developed for diabetes and analgesic management of surgical patients.

Teaching Clinical Oral and Maxillofacial Surgery

There are several well-established methods for teaching any subject. These include didactic lectures, in person or via Zoom, discussion and videos of surgical procedures, small group learning, problem-based learning, competency based, narrative, and so forth. Overall, clinical learning can be patient-based, animal-based, or simulation-based.[10,11]

Didactic Programs and Clinical Programs

An interesting article[12] followed the 3-year impact of teaching integrated dental alveolar surgery via problem-based learning on graduates. In a 72-hour course, replacement of 62 hours of didactic lectures with 60 hours of problem-based discussion, after 2 hours of preparation, had a positive impact on learning and later practice. Problem-based methods focus student attention on the problem at hand and help direct learning.

The numbers game is less important than assessment of students during clinical encounters. At our institution, the number of extractions required is only 5 but with full-time faculty and several rotation experiences in oral surgery and hospital dentistry, this is always exceeded. A very recent survey looked at predoctoral surgical requirements in US dental schools.[13] Periodontal surgery observation was included with the oral surgery experiences complicating the results. I mentioned full-time faculty, and this is important. Frequently, the predoctoral program suffers from inadequate teachers both in number and/or in training and preparation. Most nonprivate office oral and maxillofacial surgeons would prefer to be hospital based than school based. This is related to salary support, variety of cases, and so forth. Through many years of conferences and reports,[14] we, as a profession, have examined and discussed ways to improve dental education. Yet, very few actionable items have resulted. In our specialty, the dual degree program was a natural extension of increasing the length of residency training from 1 to 4 years. It was designed to enhance general surgical experience but not increase full-time OMFSs based in dental schools who are dedicated to student learning and not operating room cases. This is the goal of the current discussion. What can we learn from the dual degree experience? First, applicants to these programs now take the National Board of Medical Examiners Comprehensive Basic Science examination. How does this compare with the standard or new dental student achievement examinations? Although there are articles comparing Medical College Aptitude Test (MCAT) and dental apititude test (DAT), I know of no scholarly articles comparing the 2 examinations. Additionally, there has been a call for transitioning from Commission on Dental Accreditation (CODA) to the Accreditation Council for Graduate Medical Education Standards of academic productivity.[15]

Important Reports

I suggest we develop a workforce of OMFS dedicated to teaching integrated oral health and medicine to dental students to lead the effort to put the mouth back in the body. Ever since the 1995 IOM Report Dental Education at the Crossroads, followed by the first ever Surgeon General's Report calling oral disease an epidemic, to American Dental Edjucation Assoication (ADEA's) Commission on Change and Innovation efforts and most recently the 21st Century Gies Report in 2017, hardly any suggested actionable items for change have been implemented. The follow-up Surgeon General's Report was delayed and finally released in late 2021 by the national Institute of Dental and Craniofacial Research (NIDCR). We must use this COVID-induced time of transition in dental education and practice for substantive adaptive change. A. LeRoy Johnson the Dean of the Harvard Dental School when it changed its name to the Harvard School of Dental Medicine (1940–45) said in his small but insightful book, Dentistry as I See It, "dentistry is the only profession where the degree is awarded before professional competency is achieved".[16] Experimentation in dental education is just as important as more research on oral health and disease. Why was the Harvard School of Dental Medicine such a challenge to organized dentistry in the 1940s yet the model for Univesity of California Los Angeles (UCLA), Universityh of Conneticut (UCONN), and Stony Brook's new schools?

The list of articles promoting change for dental education just from the time of the Institute of Medicine (IOM) study in 1995 is breathtaking. All of these highlight the increasing need to improve access to care, reduce health disparities, help deal with an aging population with multiple chronic diseases, and modulate increasing health-care costs. There is increasing support for making oral health part of primary care medicine.[17] Most reforms fail to move beyond the denial or resistance stages, particularly when they are not provoked by a galvanizing event. Might the pandemic be such an event?

Improving the medical curriculum in predoctoral dental education is a priority goal of the AAOMS Committee on Predoctoral Education and Training.[18] The Pandemic has slowed us down but we must regroup in order to bypass the enemies of innovation that exist in our profession. We need adaptive change not technical change, and that always involves a loss for some group.[19]

Let us examine the recommendations of the AAOMS Committee on Predoctoral Education and Training proposed in 2017. The committee believes dentistry will have to assume a path that is more convergent with than divergent from medicine.[4,20]

Dental patient needs and potential therapies of the future will require more knowledge and skills in clinical medicine and biomedical sciences, not less. Graduates need to be good technicians and surgeons but also thoughtful health-care professionals. We need to be cognizant of the CODA rules but not dominated by them. Some years ago, a conference of research-intensive dental schools was held. Only 27 were invited, for they in fact did research. The remaining dental schools were furious at their omission. It did lead to a CODA requirement for research. It reads, "Research, the process of scientific inquiry involved in the development and dissemination of new knowledge, must be an integral component of the purpose/mission, goals and objectives of the dental school."

I doubt it is being met completely by schools. This highlights an important issue; can innovation overcome incumbency. CODA rules do not change professional culture.

Some new methods of teaching may help. The recent 21st Century Gies Report[14] highlighted challenges facing dental schools. These include outdated financial and educational models, shrinking demand for dental services, shifting practice environment, and insufficient support for research. All of these in some way emphasize the need for increasing integration with medical and other health profession schools. This pandemic has impacted that. If we recall, the HIV AIDS epidemic, led to all of us wearing gloves. Hard to believe, we didn't do that that before 1982. What might the COVID pandemic bring to our profession? It certainly has led some broadening of scope in terms of dentists giving vaccination but organized dentistry still refrains from supporting oral health in Medicare, and sees dentists as vaccinators as a major success in changing scope. How about checking blood pressures, checking for oral cancers, and so forth. A few years ago, the American Dental Association (ADA) advised dentists to be advocates for human papilloma virus (HPV) vaccination to prevent cervical and oral pharyngeal cancers. Why did not they advise dentists to give the vaccinations without the threat of a pandemic?

Why have not I mentioned predoctoral surgical requirements in US dental schools? In fact, a recent article examined this considering changes due to the COVID-19 pandemic. This survey-based study[13] suggested that as of 2020, only a small fraction of US dental programs require surgical experiences. Periodontal surgical observation via assisting was counted toward surgical experience but trends noted were more surgical experiences in east coast schools, and a more robust surgical experience in a program with a small class size. Clearly, COVID has affected this.

What about didactic curriculum. Dental graduates should know about impactions, cysts, tumors, and so forth. Identification and referral for oral cancers is a critical skill for predoctoral dental students. The method of teaching can vary but student involvement via group learning, problem-based learning, and especially person-centered approach can transform dental education. There must be a shift toward teaching and learning in the predoctoral school environment, by well-prepared faculty who are adequately supported to be full time. Prepared faculty can use the example of the odontogenic keratocyst to teach about the sonic hedgehog pathway, and current research on ameloblastoma can illuminate and make basic science so relevant. Clinical identification of oral factors is of utmost importance but there is much that can be included in an oral cancer discussion on general development of malignancy and its understanding. William Gies lamented in his classic report[21] that dentistry and dental education in 1926 was mechanical, empiric, commercial, reparative, and isolated from other disciplines. Research he said had been almost exclusively mechanical and only incidentally biological. Is this not the continuing problem?

Attention to predoctoral education by oral and maxillofacial surgery and all our educational institutions and teachers can make a difference in the scope and practice of oral health in general. Removal of teeth needs to be learned but the stimulation of the mind is critical. "The key to reform of almost any kind in higher education lies not in the way that knowledge is produced. It lies in the way that the producers of knowledge are produced."[22]

REFERENCES

1. Gordon S, Donoff RB. Problems and solutions for interprofessional education in North American dental schools. Dent Clin North Am 2016;60(4):811–24.
2. Hendricson W, Cohen PA. Oral health care in the 21st century; implications for dental and medical education. Acad Med 2001;76(12):1181–206.
3. Donoff RB, Daley GQ. Oral health care in the 21st century: I is time for integration of dental and medical education. J Dent Educ 2020;84(9):999–1002.
4. Quock RL, Al-Sabbagh M, Mason MK, et al. The dentists as doctor: a rallying call for the future. Oral Surg Oral Med Oral Pathol Oral Radiol 2014;118:637–41.
5. Donoff RB, McDonough JE, Riedy CA. Integrating oral and general health care. N Engl J Med 2014;371:2247–9.
6. Watt RG, Serban S. Multimorbidity: a challenge and opportunity for the dental profession. Br Dent J 2020;229:282–6.
7. Savageau JA, Sullivan K, Hargraves JL, et al. Oral health curriculum evaluation tool (OHCET) for

primary care training programs. J Dent Educ 2021; 85:1710–7.

8. Majprivez C, et al. Management of dental extractions in patients undergoing anticoagulant oral direct treatment: a pilot study. Oral Surg Oral Med Oral Pathol 2016;122:e146–55.

9. Yoshikawa H. Safety of tooth extraction in patients receiving direct oral anticoagulant treatment versus warfarin: a prospective observation study. Int J Oral Maxillofac Surg 2019;48:1102–8.

10. Lund B, et al. Student perception of two different simulation techniques in oral and maxillofacial surgery undergraduate training. BMC Med Educ 2011;11:82.

11. Feng J, Qi W, Duan S, et al. Three-dimensional printed model of impacted third molar for surgical extraction training. J Dent Educ 2021;85:1828–36.

12. Bai X, Kiaofeng B, et al. Follow-up assessment of problem-based learning in dental alveolar surgery education: a pilot trial. Int Dental J 2017;67:180–5.

13. Bello SA, Ray N, Shearer TR, et al. A Descriptive analysis of predoctoral surgical requirements in US dental schools in 2020. J Dent Ed 2021;1–10. https://doi.org/10.1002/jdd12832.

14. Formicola AJ, et al. Advancing dental education in the 21st century: phase 2 report on strategic analysis and recommendations. J Dental Education 2018;82: es 1.

15. Jazayert HE, Chuang SK. Transitioning from commission on dental accreditation to accreditation council for graduate medical education standards of academic productivity: a new paradigm. J Oral Maxillofac Surg 2018;76:183501836.

16.. Johnson AL. Dentistry-as I see it today. New York: Little Brown and Co; 1955.

17. The Primary Care Collaborative. Innovations in oral health and primary care integration: alignment with the shared principles of primary care. 2021. Available at. https://www.pcpcc.org/resource/innovations-oral-health-and-primary-care-integration-alignment-shared-principles.

18. Dennis MJ, Bennet JD, DeLuke DE, et al. Improving the medical curriculum in predoctoral dental education: recommendations from the american association of oral and maxillofacial surgeons committee on predoctoral education and training. J Oral Maxillofac Surg 2016;75(2):240–4.

19. Heifetz RA, Linsky M. Leadership on the LIne: staying alive through the dangers of leading. Boston, MA: Harvard Business School Press; 2002.

20. Dennis MJ. Predoctoral dental education and the fuiture of oral and maxillofacial surgery. J Oral Maxillofac Surg 2011;69:248–51.

21. Donoff RB. The Gies report and research. J Am Coll Dent 2002;69(2):22–5.

22.. Menand L. The marketplace of ideas. reform and resistance in the American university. Boston, MA: W. W. Norton and Company; 2010. p. 157.

Oral and Maxillofacial Surgery Training in the United States

Influences of Dental and Medical Education, Wartime Experiences, and Other External Factors

Leonard B. Kaban, DMD, MD[a],*, Robert Hale, DDS[b],
David H. Perrott, DDS, MD, MBA, FACS[c]

KEYWORDS

- Oral and maxillofacial surgery training ● OMS Residency programs ● History ● Training programs

KEY POINTS

- Dental Surgery training apprenticeships.
- Mid-20th century ABOMS established.
- Mid-20th century integrated 3 year and then 4-year programs.
- 1970s dual degree programs.
- Military Contributions.

INTRODUCTION

In the 19th century, surgical care was primitive; operations were infrequent and, of necessity, carried out with lightning speed. Mortality rates were exceedingly high. The variables of pain, hemorrhage, shock, and infection were the major obstacles to successful outcomes, patient survival, and advancement of the discipline of surgery.

In this article, we trace the history of education and training of oral and maxillofacial surgeons as it evolved, from apprenticeships in the mid-19th century to the present, in parallel with advances in surgery. We consider the effects of separation of medicine and dentistry, the discovery of ether anesthesia, antisepsis, and antibiotics and wars had on surgical progress, expansion of scope, and evolution of training. Finally, we describe the interest in pursuing a postresidency medical degree by individual surgeons after World War II and the subsequent development of the dual degree OMS paradigm in the 1970s.

19th century oral and maxillofacial surgery

Surgical training in the 19th century

In the early 1800s, the most common dental surgical operation was tooth extraction. Dental and physician surgeons also debrided wounds, excised tumors, drained neck space infections, and treated pain by nerve transection or neurectomy. In addition, nonhealthcare providers, for example, barbers, blacksmiths who apprenticed to established surgeons (MDs), or dental

[a] Walter C. Guralnick Distinguished Professor &Chief Emeritus, Department of Oral & Maxillofacial Surgery, Massachusetts General Hospital, Harvard School of Dental Medicine, Boston, MA 02114, USA; [b] U.S. Army, 6325 Topanga Canyon Rd, Suite 435, Woodland Hills, CA 91367, USA; [c] California Hospital Association, Phoenix, CA, USA
* Corresponding author. Department of OMS, Massachusetts General Hospital, 55 Fruit Street, Boston, MA 02114.
E-mail address: kaban.leonard@mgh.harvard.edu

Oral Maxillofacial Surg Clin N Am 34 (2022) 495–503
https://doi.org/10.1016/j.coms.2022.03.008

surgeons, also did these procedures. There were no dental schools; medical schools existed, but they had no strict entry requirements. As we know them today, government regulations or oversight, analytical clinical studies, or evidence-based medicine principles were not available to guide practice.[1,2] There were no formal institutional training programs for surgeons. Therefore, physicians, who chose to do so, apprenticed to well-known dental or general surgeons.

Events that had a significant impact on oral surgery beginning in the 19th century

Discovery of ether anesthesia The demonstration of ether at Massachusetts General Hospital (MGH), in October 1846,[3–5] was followed later by solutions to the other major barriers to the successful advancement of surgical care: (1) antisepsis described by Joseph Lister in 1867[6,7], (2) antibiotics and the discovery of Penicillin by Alexander Fleming in 1928[8], (3) transplantation, the first human organ transplant in 1955[9,10], and (4) advances in fluid and electrolyte management.[11] This progression of milestones and advances, beginning in the 19th century, allowed surgical treatment to evolve in stages from excision/ablation only, to reconstruction, transplantation, induction, and regeneration, to its current state.[2,12]

The discovery of anesthesia is particularly relevant to surgical training because it allowed surgeons to do complex operations, paying careful attention to precise execution, without the patient thrashing about in pain. This facilitated the development of more extensive and complicated surgical techniques which, in turn, necessitated expanded and more sophisticated education for the modern surgeon.

The role of dental surgeons was critical in the demonstration and dissemination of ether anesthesia. William Morton, Horace Wells, and Nathan Cooley Keep, 3 dentists, recognized the importance and significance of discovering a technique to alleviate pain and suffering caused by dental and surgical procedures.[3] At that time, most medical care was delivered in patients' homes or surgeons' offices and not in the hospital. They immediately recognized the efficiency and utility of out-patient surgery with "etherization." After the initial demonstration of ether, Keep hired Morton, and they advertised their practice of "painless dentistry" in the local newspapers. This ultimately led to the surgeon/anesthetist model that has defined American Oral and Maxillofacial Surgery in the 20th and 21st centuries and has significantly influenced the curriculum and clinical training of oral and maxillofacial surgeons.[2,3]

Formation of a university affiliated and degree-granting dental school Another major event in the mid-19th century (1867) was the formation of a university-affiliated and degree-granting dental school, Harvard School of Dental Medicine. This was established because Harvard University did not wish to award the MD degree to students of dentistry. Baltimore Dental College, a nonuniversity affiliated school, was established earlier. The 2 schools provided the opportunity for a practitioner with a DDS (Baltimore) or DMD (Harvard) degree to practice dental surgery. Dentistry and dental surgery were effectively separated from medicine, a dichotomy that has prevailed to this day and has had a profound impact on oral surgery training. In 1971, 104 years later, it is ironic that the same Medical School and University approved a program to finally award Oral and Maxillofacial Surgeons an MD degree as their "lawful appendage."[2]

The American civil war Progress was made in the Civil War in the general management of combat casualties and hemorrhage. For the first time, there were advances in battlefield anesthesia (after the discovery of ether). A series of hospitals to take progressive care of the wounded, antisepsis, sanitation, and advances in nursing care were introduced to improve control of hemorrhage and prevent infection. These changes had a positive impact on the survival of the injured combatants.[13] (**Table 1**). In dental surgery, James Baxter Bean and Thomas Brian Gunning first described the use of dental splints to help reduce and immobilize jaw fractures.[14]

Late 19th, early 20th century changes in the specialty In the late 19th century, building on the advances mentioned above, the evolution of OMS progressed because oral surgeons and their organizations appreciated the need to improve education, training, and standards of practice.[15] As the 19th-century exodontists (physicians, dentists, barbers, other nonprofessionals) expanded the field in the early 20th century, they changed the specialty and organizational names to reflect these increases in the knowledge base and scope of clinical practice: American Society of Exodontists (1918), American Society of Exodontists and Oral Surgeons (1921), This evolution, in turn, led to adaptive changes in the training of oral surgeons.[15–18]

Contributions of 20th and 21st century wars on the training of oral and maxillofacial surgery Progress in general surgical care and advances in OMS continued through World Wars I and II, Korean and Vietnam wars. The advances included

Table 1
MMR and supporting RMMAs

MMR	RMMA
Wound care and patient transport, 16–18th centuries	Dressings and abandonment of hot oil(Pair) Gunpowder not a poison (Hunter) Flying ambulance (Larrey) Hospital as a sanctuary(Pringle)
19th century (American Civil War, Franco-Prussian War, Crimean War)	Hospital systems Anesthesia Antisepsis/sanitation (Lister, Pateur, Koch) Nursing care (Nightingale)
World War I and World War II	Antibiotics Blood transfusions Dakin's solution Positive-pressure ventilation for "wet lung" Traction for femur fractures
Korean War and Vietnam War	Renal dialysis Helicopter evacuation Transcontinental evacuation Vascular repair Mafenide burn topical Identification of acute respiratory distress syndrome ("Da Nand lung")

Abbreviations: MMR, military medical revolution; RMMA, Revolution in Military Medical Affairs.
Adapted from Pruitt BA, Pruitt JH. History of trauma care. In: Feliciano D, Mattox J, Moore E, eds. Trauma. 6th ed. McGraw-Hill, New York: Medical; 2008:1Y23.

improvements in the general care of the injured patient, resuscitation, hemorrhage, wound care, and technical and surgical improvements in the management of craniomaxillofacial trauma.

The more recent conflicts in Iran and Afghanistan are differentiated from previous wars by the large numbers of casualties inflicted on young men and women from missiles, shrapnel, and thermal injuries. The damage often consisted of composite tissue loss, contaminated wounds, and loss of facial subunits. Modern military medicine, forward hospital facilities, well-trained medics and corpsmen, body armor, efficient evaluation and evacuation from the battlefield, and high survivability from blood loss and shock created a challenge in modern times to manage the severe general and head and neck injuries of returning soldiers (**Table 2**).[13,19,20]

These clinical experiences have also led to considerable translational and clinical research, which has had implications for civilian patients and has increased the scope of OMS as a specialty, necessitating more sophisticated training..[13,19,20] (see **Tables 1** and **2**).

As in every war, oral and maxillofacial surgeons who served in the combat support hospitals eventually rotated home to enrich civilian and military OMS postgraduate training as faculty and invited speakers. Combat Casualty Courses centralized

at Walter Reed, Bethesda, and San Antonio Military Medical Centers have ensured that the combat theater has increasingly more trained and experienced oral and maxillofacial surgeons to fulfill its needs on the battlefield. This experience has also augmented civilian trauma and reconstructive surgery training.

Evolution of oral and maxillofacial surgery training programs

Up until the 1930s, 1-year internships, apprenticeships, "limiting practice to oral surgery" were the norms for training. Formal programs included a 1-year oral surgery internship; a second year consisting of didactic courses in anatomy, physiology, and so forth, at a dental school. This was followed by a 2nd clinical year, considered the residency, often at a different institution.[2,15–18]

In 1967, the American Society of Oral Surgeons (ASOS) Committee on Graduate Training, as a result of a number of educational workshops, recommended a revision of the Essentials of an Adequate Advanced Training Program in Oral Surgery. The new Essentials mandated a 3-year integrated program which included a 1-year oral surgery internship followed by 1 year of hospital rotations in medicine (3 months), surgery (3 months), anesthesia (3 months), and an elective

Table 2
RMMAs, 2001 to 2011 OCOs in Afghanistan and Iraq

OCO	RMMA
Deployed hospital care	DCR
	Diagnostic evaluation for explosion injury
	Vascular surgery
	Ortho wound care
	Regional anesthesia and TIVA
	Combat burn care
	Management of TBI
	Surgical intervention for penetrating TBI
	Negative-pressure combat wound dressings
	Intravenous TXA
	Far-forward MIS
	Coagulation monitoring with thromboelastography/RoTEM
En route care	Global en route care (CCATT and Burn Flight Team)
	En route critical care nursing US Army flight medic training

Abbreviations: DCR, delivery change report; OCO, overseas contingency operations; RMMA, Revolution in Military Medical Affairs.

From Blackbourne LH, Baer DG, Eastridge BJ, Renz EM, Chung KK, Dubose J, Wenke JC, Cap AP, Biever KA, Mabry RL, Bailey J, Maani CV, Bebarta VS, Rasmussen TE, Fang R, Morrison J, Midwinter MJ, Cestero RF, Holcomb JB. Military medical revolution: deployed hospital and en route care. J Trauma Acute Care Surg. 2012 Dec;73(6 Suppl 5):S378 to 87.

(3 months). The third year was the senior OMS residency experience. All programs had to provide a progression of complexity and responsibility in training at the home institution. The Commission on Dental Accreditation (CODA) approved this change.[2,15–18]

In 1985, the AAOMS House of Delegates approved a resolution to increase OMS training from 3 to 4 years. The resolution mandated that all programs follow a 4-year integrated, progressive curriculum consisting of 1-year oral surgery internship; followed by 1 year of off-service rotations (3 months medicine, 3 months surgery, 4 months anesthesia, 2 months elective) and then 24 months of OMS, 12 each at the junior and senior resident levels. CODA approved these changes in December 1986.[2,15–18] Over the years, the anesthesia requirement has increased to 5 months, including a pediatric anesthesia experience (1-month). In addition, requirements for ACLS (advanced cardiac life support), PALS (pediatric advanced life support), and scholarly activity have been instituted.

As noted above, war-time experiences and the resulting increased scope of oral surgery stimulated an interest in the development of "dual degree" training programs after WWII and through the 1970s and 80s. Subsequently, in the late 20th and early 21st centuries, advanced fellowship training programs in subspecialty areas such as head and neck cancer, cleft/craniofacial and orthognathic, pediatric maxillofacial, cosmetic, reconstructive, and temporomandibular joint (TMJ) surgery were developed.

Concurrently with this evolution, the American Board of Oral and Maxillofacial Surgery (ABOMS) improved the sophistication and standardization of the certifying examination and AAOMS developed the Oral and Maxillofacial Surgery In-Training Examination (OMSITE),[15–18] first administered in 1977, to evaluate residents as they advanced through their levels of training.

Development of the modern dual degree oral and maxillofacial surgery program: background

In the late 1960s, Dr Walter Guralnick (**Fig. 1**), Chief of Oral Surgery at Massachusetts General Hospital (MGH) and Harvard School of Dental Medicine (HSDM) and chairman of the American Society of Oral Surgeons Committee on Graduate Training (later to become Committee on Residency Education and Training, CRET) concluded that dual

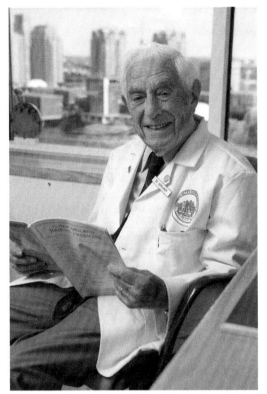

Fig. 1. Dr Walter c. Guralnick, circa 2013. (*Courtesy of* Leonard B. Kaban, DMD, MD, FACS, Boston, MA)

degree training would be important for oral and maxillofacial surgeons.

Dr Guralnick described, in an article published in JOMS in 1973[15], the rationale for the MGH/Harvard MD Oral and Maxillofacial Surgery program, which was formally proposed in 1970 and implemented in 1971. He concluded that the increasingly complex scope of OMS as a specialty required a significant change in training.[15] He made the following points: (1) "....., there is an educational deficit in oral surgery training programs consisting of insufficient general medical and surgical background." (2) This deficiency would best be corrected by "obtaining a medical degree and general surgery training, in addition to the OMS experience" (3) ".....this is consistent with the direction of our specialty and our standards of training."

He recognized that: "A major curricular change cannot be made without considerable trauma to the group affected by it."[15] James Hayward,[21] at the time editor-in-chief of Journal of Oral Surgery (JOS) and the Chairman of Oral Surgery at the University of Michigan, wrote regarding the implementation of dual degree programs: "....we fully appreciate that our particular goals in education

require the teamwork of agencies in dentistry, medicine, and hospitals."[15,22,23]

Dr Guralnick also maintained that the MD degree and at least 1 year of legitimate general surgery training would lead to a more confident and competent surgeon, better patient care, and better education for the residents. His forward thinking was also evidenced by the fact that he was one of a few OMS chiefs, at the time, to appreciate the importance of the "full-time" faculty model. In the 1960s, most OMS programs had predominantly part-time faculty whose primary responsibilities were in their private practices. Dr Guralnick was confident that dual degree training and the full-time faculty model would significantly improve the status of OMS as a specialty in the hospital and university and would allow us to be integrated into the mainstream of American Surgery.

Objections to dual degree training in the 1960s and 1970s

included: 1) Specialized OMS training might be adversely affected by shortening its length to devote time to the MD degree and general surgery residency. 2) Expense and time involved would be overwhelming and discourage potential applicants, and 3) There would be a potential for loss of residents to other specialties.[15,22,23]

It should be noted that in the 1940s through the 1970s, some pioneer oral surgeons were independently enrolling in medical school and obtaining an MD degree to enhance their training. There are no specific records identifying these OMSs, but those that we were able to document are listed in **Table 3**.[1,2]

Many of these "dual degree" oral surgeons assumed academic positions (but some had private practices on the side) and became program directors and department chairmen (see **Table 3**). Despite seeking an MD degree and general surgery training for themselves, the majority did not pursue the development of dual-degree programs at their respective institutions.[2] They may not have been allowed to pursue this goal or may not have appreciated its significance for the evolution and progress of the Specialty.

Early dual degree programs: the first 5

Harvard plan

As noted above, the Harvard Plan was conceived in the late 1960s, approved in 1970, and enrolled its first resident into the full program as written in 1971[2,15,24].

On completing the MGH/Harvard program, the resident received an OMS certificate, MD degree, credit for 2 years of general surgery, and 32 months of OMS. The key points are that postgraduate year

Table 3
Oral Surgeons who went to Medical School on their own from the 1930s–1970s

William Harrigan	DDS, University of Pennsylvania,1938; MD New York University, 1942. Chief, Bellevue Hospital, 1950.
Edward Hinds[a]	DDS, 1940; MD, 1945 Baylor University, Chairman, University of Texas Houston, 1948.
Marsh Robinson	DDS, 1942; MD, 1946, University of Southern California. Chairman, University Southern California, 1954.
Charles "Scotty" McCallum	DMD, Tufts 1952; MD, University of Alabama. 1957, Chairman UAB 1958.
Morton Goldberg	DMD, Harvard 1958; MD, Albany Medical College, 1961 Chief, Hartford Hospital, 1971.
Donald Leake[a]	DMD, Harvard 1962; MD, Stanford University 1969. Chief, Harbor UCLA Medical Center, 1970.
Victor Matukas[b]	DMD, Loyola U, New Orleans; MD University-Colorado 1968; Dept Chair University of Alabama, 1985
Norman Trieger	DMD, Harvard, 1954; MD, Albert Einstein 1974. Chief, Montefiore Medical Center, 1973.
H. David Hall[b]	DMD, Harvard, 1957; MD, University of Alabama, 1977 Chairman, University of Alabama, 1958; Chairman Vanderbilt University, 1968.
James Bird	DDS University of Nebraska 1969; MD University of Nebraska 1973.
James Bertz[a]	DDS, Ohio State University 1961; MD, Baylor University 1974.
Roger Meyer[a,c]	DDS University of Washington 1963; MD Creighton University 1975; Chair, Emory University 1979.

[a] FACS.
[b] Started dual degree program Vanderbilt (Hall), Alabama (Matukas).
[c] Received approval for a dual degree program at Emory.
From Kaban LB, Perrott DH. Dual-degree Oral and Maxillofacial Surgery Training in the United States: "Back to the Future". J Oral Maxillofac Surg. 2020 Jan;78(1):18 to 28.

(PGY)-1 was 12 months OMS, and 20 of the last 24 months were devoted to OMS. This continues to be the template for the MGH/Harvard Program and has been a model for many dual degree residencies in the United States. However, some programs cannot provide the equivalent continuity of OMS experience because the time is disrupted by medical school requirements/rotations. A summary of the current MGH/Harvard MD Program appears in **Box 1**.

A 30-year follow-up study demonstrated that the fear of loss of residents proved not to be a significant problem. Only 4 of the first 55 (7.1%) and 1 of the second 55 (1.8%) residents failed to complete the program. This compares favorably to any surgical program 6 years in length, whereby there may be loss of some residents over the long duration of training.[2,24]

The MGH program was arguably the first contemporary dual degree program accepted by its Medical School, Dental School, and the University.

University of Nebraska

Contemporaneously with the development of the MGH/Harvard dual degree program, Dr Chester Singer, Chair of OMS at the University of Nebraska Medical Center, sought to develop an MD/OMS plan. With support from the Chair of Surgery, Dr Merle Musselman, and the medical school, the 5-year dual degree program at the University of Nebraska Medical Center was approved in 1970. The first residents were enrolled in 1971. Since 1971, all residents have trained in the fully integrated dual degree program, and today the program is 6 years in duration (Personal communication: Valmont D, OMS University of Nebraska; In the late 1970s through 1981, 3 additional dual degree programs were implemented, bringing the total to 5: University of Alabama-Birmingham; Vanderbilt University; and University of Washington, Seattle. Personal communication:"Scotty" McCallum C, Robinson K, University of Alabama, Birmingham, Alabama, 2019; Personal communication: McKenna S, Chair, Department

Box 1 **MGH, Harvard MD Oral and Maxillofacial Surgery Program: Started 1971, modified 1986 and 1999, 6 years[a]**
• Current form: PGY 1, OMS Intern 12 months
• PGY 2, Harvard Medical School 3rd year
• PGY 3, Harvard Medical School 4th year
○ Four months anesthesia
• PGY 4, MGH General Surgery PGY 2
• PGY 5, MGH General Surgery
○ PGY 3, 4 months (1-month SICU)
■ OMS Junior 8 months
• PGY 6, OMS Chief Resident, 4 months
○ OMS Senior Resident, 4 months
○ Children Hospital Senior, 4 months
• First-year and 20 months of the final 24 months uninterrupted OMS
• Credit for 2 years of general Surgery
[a] Classic program as written. There will be some changes in enrollment years in medical school (eg,2nd and 3rd rather than 3rd and 4th) based on a new Harvard Medical School Curriculum, but the basic 6-year template will remain the same.
Modified from Kaban LB, Perrott DH. Dual-degree Oral and Maxillofacial Surgery Training in the United States: "Back to the Future". J Oral Maxillofac Surg. 2020 Jan;78(1):18 to 28.,

Box 2 **Current (2021–2022) OMS Program Data from AAOMS**
• Number of Accredited OMS Programs:100
• Number of Single Degree OMS Programs: 56
• Number of Dual Degree OMS Programs:44
• Number of Programs to offer single-and dual-degree tracks: 22
• Number of Hospital-based Programs: 44
• Number of Dental School-based Programs: 37
• Number of Medical School-based Programs: 9
• Number of Federal Service Programs: 10
• Current Residents in Training for 2021 to 2022: 1207
• Number of Residents in Single-degree Programs: 690 (57%)
• Number of Residents in Dual-degree Programs:517 (43%)
• Number of 2021 to 2022 available first-year positions: 236
• Number enrolled in single degree: 129 (55%)
• Number enrolled in dual degree: 106 (45%)
• Total Number of Female Residents: 254 (21%),
• Total Number of Male Residents: 953 (79%)
From American Association of Oral and Maxillofacial Surgeons Data, 2014 to 2018, 2020 to 2021.

of OMS Vanderbilt University, Nashville Tennessee, 2020; Personal communication: Joseph Piecuch, DMD, MD, Simsbury, CT, 2019)[25,26].

Current oral and maxillofacial surgery training programs

Since 1981, the total number of dual degree programs has grown, from the 5 mentioned above, to 44 of the 100 accredited American OMS programs. The 5-year trend (2014–2018) of AAOMS data for graduating residents revealed about 2/3 were in single degree and 1/3 in dual degree programs.[2] AAOMS data from 2021 to 2022 show 57% of graduates are from single degree and 43% from dual degree programs (**Box 2**.).

It is of interest that single-degree OMS postgraduate training predominates in the military for various reasons. First and foremost is that the scope of practice and capabilities are consistent with the needs of the military. As their most compelling argument, advocates for dual-degree OMS training in the military have the nearly 100% retention of dual-trained OMS surgeons for a 20-year career. There are many other advantages, but the usual reasons for a dual degree program are not nearly as operative in the military, especially because Inter-specialty competition is almost nonexistent in this setting.

American College of Surgeons
Until 2016, fellowship in the American College of Surgeons was limited to ABOMS certified dual-degree OMSs who went through a complex double-tiered admission process. Edward Hinds, DDS, MD, was the first OMS to become a fellow in the ACS. However, he was board-certified in general surgery. The first nongeneral surgeon OMS admitted to fellowship was Dr Donald Leake (1974) and, thereafter, Dr Leonard Kaban (1980). In 1990, the next 3 OMSs admitted were Drs James Bertz, R. Bruce Donoff, and Harry Schwartz. As many as 45 to 50 dual-degree OMSs became fellows over the years through this process. In 2016, the American College of Surgeons (ACS), working with Dr Ghali Ghali and a special committee of AAOMS, simplified the admission process for

dual degree OMSs. Soon after that, a pathway for single-degree OMSs to attain fellowship was established. The number of fellows dramatically increased to more than 200, and an OMS section was established, with Steven Roser as its Chair. Oral and Maxillofacial Surgeons joined the mainstream of American Surgery as Dr Guralnick predicted.

DISCUSSION

Multiple factors have contributed to the evolution and growth of the modern specialty of OMS. These have included experiences in the management of severe traumatic injuries during wartime. remarkable advances in biomedical sciences, surgical technique, and instrumentation; imaging; anesthetic drugs and techniques; improvements in education and teaching; measuring outcomes of training; the full-time faculty model in tertiary care medical centers and dual-degree residency programs.

The dual-degree concept has truly changed the "face" of OMS. It has also contributed to the development of advanced training fellowships in head and neck and reconstructive, cleft/craniofacial/pediatric, cosmetic, and TMJ surgery. As predicted by Walter Guralnick, in his early writings, the MD degree, general surgery training, full-time faculty model, and a broader scope have resulted in wide acceptance of OMS as a surgical specialty by universities, medical schools, and hospitals. It is not uncommon now for ENT, Plastic Surgery, and General Surgery residents to rotate on OMS services during their early years. This allows them to gain familiarity, knowledge, and respect for our field.

The full-time faculty model has also integrated OMS into the Medical Centers where we function and where many OMS faculty have come to occupy leadership positions. All this has led to the acceptance of ABOMS certification as a credential for fellowship eligibility in the ACS. Four Oral and Maxillofacial Surgeons have been Chairmen of the JCAHO (Charles McCallum, DMD, MD, John Helfrick DDS, David Whiston, DDS, and David Perrott, DDS, MD, MBA, FACS).

Despite all the progress, there are challenges ahead, including but not limited to: (1) changes in medical school curricula, making it more difficult to find a natural place for OMS transfer students; (2) increasing time OMS residents have to spend in medical school to avoid diluting the OMS experience; (3) growing number of years of ACGME accredited postgraduate training requirements for medical licensure; (4) increasing cost of education; (5) decreasing reimbursement for OMS

services by government payors and insurance companies. In addition, there is expanding competition from overlapping dental and medical/surgical specialties in OMS areas of practice, for example, dental implants, orthognathic surgery, and reconstructive surgery. The authors suggest that care should be taken to develop innovative programs to resolve the above problems without significantly increasing the 6-year template. We are optimistic that satisfactory innovative solutions will be achieved and that the future will be bright for OMS.

ACKNOWLEDGMENTS

There is not a significant written record of the evolution of Oral and Maxillofacial Surgery training in the United States. In particular, the development of dual degree programs is not well documented in the literature. Therefore, the information we obtained from conversations with, emails, and letters from the following surgeons was invaluable in completing this study: Drs Samuel McKenna, Peter Waite, Thomas Dodson, Morton Goldberg, James Hupp, Bruce Donoff, Ghali Ghali, Charles "Scotty" McCallum, Roger Meyer, Robert Mraule, Valmont Desa, Joseph Piecuch, John Helfrick, and Ms Kitty Robinson. We thank them for their help and encouragement. We thank Barbara Kaban for critiquing this article and helping to organize the material.

REFERENCES

1. Kaban L.B., History of dual degree training in the United States: "Back, to the future". Presented at ROAAOMS Symposium at the 100th Meeting of the American Association of Oral and Maxillofacial Surgeons, 8-13, October, 2018.

2. Kaban LB, Perrott DH. Dual-degree oral and maxillofacial surgery training in the united states: "Back to the future". J Oral Maxillofac Surg 2020;78(1):18–28.

3. Guralnick WC, Kaban LB. Keeping ether "En-Vogue": the role of nathan cooley keep in the history of ether anesthesia. J Oral Maxillofac Surg 2011;69: 1892–7.

4. Bigelow HJ. Insensibility during surgical operations produced by inhalation. Boston Med Surg J 1846; 35:309–31.

5. Keep NC. Inhalation of ethereal vapor for mitigating human suffering in surgical operations and acute diseases. Boston Med Surg J 1847;36:199–201.

6. Lister J. On a new method of treating compound fracture, abscess, &c., with observations on the conditions of 'suppuration. Lancet 1867;336–9.

7. Lister J. Further evidence regarding the effects of the antiseptic system of treatment upon the salubrity of a surgical 'hospital. Lancet 1870;287–8.

8. Fleming A. On the antibacterial action of cultures of a penicillium, with special reference to their use in the isolation of B. influenzae. Br J Exp Pathol 1929; 10:226–36.

9. Murray JE, Merrill JP, Harrison JH. Renal homotransplantation in identical twins. Surg Forum 1956;6: 432–6.

10. Merrill JP, Murray JE, Harrison JH, et al. Successful homotransplantations of the human kidney between identical twins. J Amer Med Assoc 1956;160: 277–82.

11. Moore FD. Metabolic care of the surgical patient. Philadelphia and London: W. B. Saunders Co.; 1959.

12. Murray JE: Presidential address Boston surgical society. 1979, Boston, MA.

13. Dodson TB, Guralnick WC, Donoff RB, et al. Massachusetts general hospital/harvard medical school md oral & maxillofacial surgery program: a 30-year review. J Oral Maxillofac Surg 2004;62:62–5.

14. Blackbourne LH, Baer DG, Eastridge BJ, et al. Military medical revolution: prehospital combat casualty care. J Trauma Acute Care Surg 2012;73(6 Suppl 5): S372–7. Erratum in: J Trauma Acute Care Surg. 2013 Feb;74(2):705. Kotwal, Russell S [corrected to Kotwal, Russ S]. Erratum in: J Trauma Acute Care Surg. 2013 Jan;74(1):347.

15. Pollock RA. Management of jaw injuries in the American civil war: the diuturnity of bean in the South, gunning in the north. Craniomaxillofac Trauma Reconstr 2011;4(2):85–90.

16. Guralnick WC. The combined oral surgery-MD program: the Harvard plan. J Oral Surg 1973;31:271–6.

17. Alling CC, Hayward JR. The building of a specialty: Oral & Maxillofacial Surgery in the United States, 1918-1998. A Suppl J Oral Maxillofacial Surg 1998; 69-73:165–8.

18. Alling CC, Hayward JR. The building of a specialty: Oral & Maxillofacial Surgery in the United States, 1918-1998. A Suppl J Oral Maxillofacial Surg 1998; 120–1.

19. Alling CC, Hayward JR. The building of a specialty: Oral & Maxillofacial Surgery in the United States, 1918-1998. A Suppl J Oral Maxillofacial Surg 1998; 287–8.

20. Blackbourne LH, Baer DG, Eastridge BJ, et al. Military medical revolution: deployed hospital and en route care. J Trauma Acute Care Surg 2012;73(6 Suppl 5):S378–87. Erratum in: J Trauma Acute Care Surg. 2013 Feb;74(2):705. Bebarta, Vikhyat [corrected to Bebarta, Vikhyat S]. PMID: 23192059.

21. Blackbourne LH, Baer DG, Eastridge BJ, et al. Military medical revolution: military trauma system. J Trauma Acute Care Surg 2012;73(6 Suppl 5): S388–94. Erratum in: J Trauma Acute Surg. 2013 Feb;74(2):705. Kotwal, Russell S [corrected to Kotwal, Russ S]. PMID:23192060.

22. Simpson DA, David DJ. Herbert moran memorial lecture. world war i: the genesis of craniomaxillofacial surgery? ANZ J Surg 2004;74(1–2):71–7.

23. Hayward JR. Strains on a bridging specialty. J Oral Surg 1971;29:837.

24. Shira RB. The specialty of oral surgery: present and future. J Oral Surg 1969;27(4):386–94.

25. Waite PD. The university of Alabama oral & Maxillofacial surgery program. J Oral Maxillofac Surg 2007;65:3–5.

26. American Association of Oral and Maxillofacial Surgeons Data, 2014-2018, 2020-2021. Available at: AAOMS.org

Development of Competencies in Oral and Maxillofacial Surgery Training

R. John Tannyhill III, DDS, MD

KEYWORDS

- Competency • Surgical training • Operative skills • Autonomy • Competency-based education
- Residency

KEY POINTS

- Progressive resident autonomy has undergone significant modification in an era of increased attending oversight, work hour restrictions, patient safety considerations, and increased medico-legal risk.
- Traditional methods of surgical training require modification to allow for the development of both technical and nontechnical competencies.
- Innovation in simulation, surgical curricula, assessment methods, and improved technical and didactic educational models are necessary for the future development of competent graduate surgeons and excellent patient outcomes.

INTRODUCTION

Oral and maxillofacial surgery is a highly technical and demanding specialty. The demand on surgical trainees to acquire the necessary skills is a constant challenge. The goal of all graduate surgical education is to ensure that the graduate is competent to practice in his or her chosen specialty. The evaluation of a resident's competency to practice, however, has never been clearly defined, nor has the fixed period of time given for residency training in each specialty been shown to be the right amount of time for every resident to achieve competency.[1] Since the time of Halsted, the overarching paradigm in surgical training has been based on an apprenticeship model in which learning occurs within the operating room with subjective assessment methods.[2,3] It can be argued that the existing surgical educational system, before recent reductions in operative exposure and resident independence, has been producing competent surgeons for generations. However, a closer look at the literature demonstrates the need for introspection. Reports that adverse surgical events account for two-thirds of all adverse events are only surpassed by data suggesting that half are preventable and that technical faults are responsible for most of the errors.[4–6] These data, along with an increase in public and political expectations, have led to the development of strategies to improve surgical proficiency and effectiveness of training.[3] Training and progression depend on a variety of cases, workload, and subjective assessment by faculty but, with understandable changes in health care such as the reduction in working hours, pressures on operating room efficiency, and the ethical considerations of training on patients, this now needs to be reconsidered.[7]

This monograph will describe competency in the context of Oral and Maxillofacial Surgery training, discuss ways in which we currently and might possibly assess competency in the future, and suggest items we need to consider as surgical educators. Many other surgical specialties are much further down the road in reconsidering surgical training in the modern era. It is the author's hope that many of the questions posed will result in innovative and "out-of-the-box" thinking by those of us in residency programs who train and mentor the next generation of Oral and Maxillofacial Surgeons.

Massachusetts General Hospital, Harvard School of Dental Medicine, Boston, MA, USA
E-mail address: rjtannyhill@mgh.harvard.edu

Oral Maxillofacial Surg Clin N Am 34 (2022) 505–513
https://doi.org/10.1016/j.coms.2022.03.012
1042-3699/22/© 2022 Elsevier Inc. All rights reserved.

WHAT IS COMPETENCY?

Competency, in a surgical context, may be defined as the knowledge, skills, and abilities required for safe and independent practice. Often, there is overlap in of each of these areas. For instance, the ability to evaluate a patient in a clinical setting and make appropriate management decisions requires more than just technical skills. It also requires many nontechnical or "soft" skills, such as interpersonal skills, conscientiousness, recognition of limits, curiosity, and confidence. In the surgical literature, there are few studies involving the direct observation of surgical residents in a clinic setting. As educators, we continue to seek objective evidence in defining resident competence in the clinic and in all settings.

CURRENT METHODS OF ASSESSING COMPETENCY

Assessment of resident competence is a lofty goal of increasingly greater importance in an era of less operative and clinical resident independence. From a practical standpoint, ACGME (Accreditation Council for Graduate Medical Education)-based residencies are more time-based with expected subjective "milestones" rather than case numbers as a guide for program directors. Dental specialties, such as Oral and Maxillofacial Surgery, tend to have a minimal time limit (currently 48 months in OMFS) as well, but are more focused on the numbers of procedures for program completion. For example, the Commission on Dental Accreditation (CODA) Standards for OMFS 2021 sets a minimum required "first-assist" operating room cases in the final year of residency for graduation from an accredited OMFS program in 4 specific areas. Standard 4 to 11 states: For each authorized final year resident position, residents must perform 175 major oral and maxillofacial surgery procedures on adults and children, documented by at least a formal operative note. For the above 175 procedures, there must be at least 20 procedures in each category of surgery. The categories of major surgery are defined as: (1) trauma, (2) pathology, (3) orthognathic surgery, and (4) reconstructive and cosmetic surgery. Sufficient variety in each category, as specified below, must be provided.[8] So, if 10 maxillary and 10 mandibular osteotomies are completed, then the resident has met the requirements under "orthognathic surgery." Once all categories are completed with 20 or more cases and the total reaches 175 cases, the resident has accomplished the objective requirements under "Major Surgery" for graduation from a residency program, as long as the program director believes the subjective criteria are met. This introduces other potential issues, however. The term "first assist" in operative notes can be used loosely. The actual performance of the resident or contribution to the operation is not reflected in the resident's logbook that is submitted for board certification and hospital credentialing. It is simply a record of attendance and participation at a certain level in the operation. It may be confirmed by the operative note, but the actual role played by the first assist in any operation can vary based on resident experience and perceived competence as well as attending preference and is usually not documented for each step of the operation. In previous studies, resident logbooks have been found to be inaccurate in determining a resident's ability to independently practice. Recording clinical experience may be influenced by bias associated with self-reporting: delayed update, transcriptional errors, and misreporting due to inaccurate recall.[9]

Along with minimal required numbers of OR cases and anesthetic cases, the current appraisal of the knowledge base of OMFS trainees is often limited to the assessment of theoretic knowledge by multiple-choice questions through the yearly OMSITE (Oral and Maxillofacial Surgery In-service Training Examination),[10] administered by the American Board of Oral and Maxillofacial Surgery, and medical pimping.[11] Structured multiple-choice questions are generally objective and fair as individual questions can be validated and standardized.[12] Pimping, though not standardized, enables the questioner to assess trainee reasoning and surgical knowledge while under pressure as well as gauging the process by which they arrive at a decision. There is currently no stage throughout American OMFS surgical training whereby there is a formal or objective appraisal of a trainee surgeon's technical ability. Rather, the assessment of a resident's technical proficiency has been largely based on the subjective opinion of faculty, often acquired during unsystematic observations and fraught with bias and inconsistency. The additional maintenance of a written or electronic operative logbook fails to indicate the quality of the trainee's performance or the specific involvement of the trainee.[12] Both methods lack validity and are unable to consistently assess a surgical trainee's capability.[13] What about outcomes? When retrospectively used as markers for postoperative success, morbidity and mortality data are influenced by patient characteristics and a number of other hospital-specific factors and are consequently not a good indication of surgical competence.[14]

It has been shown that exposure to a wide variety of patients and clinical problems, the management of critically ill patients, resident continuity of care, and residents being given responsibility for critical management decisions are all important contributing factors in the development of confidence in a surgical trainee.[15–17] With the clinical experience of surgical residents of all specialties now limited by work hours and resident autonomy continuing to decrease, concern has grown about the confidence and competence of surgical trainees in their clinical decision-making and operative skills.[18] Other authors have demonstrated that the technical skill of a surgeon results in better patient outcomes; better technical skill scores, assessed via intraoperative video, were statistically significantly associated with lower rates of any complication, unplanned reoperation, and death or serious morbidity.[19]

How do we know that a resident has conducted enough cases of a certain procedure to be competent to safely begin independent practice? Demonstration of minimum case numbers per CODA Standards has long been one of the essential metrics to assess resident experience and competence. However, studies suggest that operative experience during residency does not correlate with self-reported competency by surgical graduates.[20] Does every resident require the same number of repetitions to be considered competent? Are those skills translatable to future advances in surgical technique; that is, if a resident is competent to perform a certain procedure, will that skillset translate to a different, but similar operation? What about those procedures with minimal exposure that fall under a specialty-specific blanket "scope of practice" from a credentialing standpoint when privileges are sought at a community hospital? Does every trainee learning curve have the same slope? In a surgical context, a learning curve can be defined as a graphic representation showing the relationship between experience with a procedure and outcome. Surgical learning curves raise interesting ethical questions regarding proper consent for resident surgeons and prompt a search for ways to simulate the operating room experience to hasten the learning curve before operating on live patients. Studies demonstrate that learning curves generally "flatten out" as experience increases, resulting in fewer complications. In addition to the lack of regulatory oversight, it is this learning curve that gives rise to many ethical and legal dilemmas.[21]

Is competency in a surgical residency limited to knowledge base and surgical skills alone? To guide medical residency training programs, the Accreditation Council for Graduate Medical Education (ACGME) has outlined 6 competencies for all residency programs to emphasize: clinical care, medical knowledge, practice-based learning and improvement, systems-based care, communication, and professionalism (**Table 1**). Just like a standardized physical examination may use an anatomic approach, these 6 competencies provide a systematic framework to think about both curriculum and assessment in residency education.

How do we determine when trainees have become proficient in specific required technical and nontechnical skills? How do we guide the development of competence through feedback? Currently, many programs use aggregate assessments from the faculty to find out when trainees have become proficient enough to practice independently. Through the AAOMS-developed "Benchmarks" and CODA Standards, minimum goals and requirements related to oral and maxillofacial surgery have been developed. However, optimal objective methods for assessing resident performance have yet to be established. Usually, assessment and feedback are conducted informally, but overall, there is a lack of objective measures in OMFS training programs. When considering available tools for the evaluation of surgical skills, we should be mindful of both formative and summative assessments. Formative assessment (assessment *for* learning) is carried out throughout the training process to allow trainees to measure and monitor their progression and continue to improve their performance. This also encourages training to be tailored to the learners' specific needs. Formative assessment must become more fully and meaningfully integrated into all aspects of training and used to enhance the learning process through timely and constructive feedback to trainees.[22] It is to provide near-immediate feedback and aid in resident learning. Tools such as the SIMPL (System for Improving and Measuring Procedural Learning) mobile phone application, which is based on the Zwisch[23] scale, has been successfully used to assess and give formative feedback on intraoperative performance in oral and maxillofacial surgery[24] as well as many other surgical specialties.[25] Summative assessment (assessment *of* learning) is typically carried out upon the completion of training and allows for accreditation and certification. For example, a summative assessment at the end of residency is completed by the program director, and the resident is certified as capable of independent practice. The establishment and implementation of ideal evaluation tools for both formative and summative

Table 1	
Six ACGME Competencies with examples of each category	
Competency	**Example**
Clinical Care	Resident-Faculty debriefing after patient care encounters; feedback after OR
Medical Knowledge	Cadaver laboratory, didactic curriculum
Practice-based Learning	Coding course, QI projects
Systems-based Care	Resident-led Morbidity and Mortality conferences; online complication reporting system
Communication	Wellness initiatives; debriefing after patient encounters
Professionalism	Professionalism-based case encounters

assessment are essential to ensuring the advancement of surgical education.[26] It is this author's opinion that our focus should remain solely on improving formative assessment methods and tools. When the summative assessment is completed, the time has passed to modify trainee behaviors or knowledge base and allow for improvement.

Miller[27] outlined a practical framework for the assessment of clinical skills, performance, and ultimately competence (**Fig. 1**). While the first 3 levels, Knows, Knows How, and Shows How, are important assessment approaches, residency programs should place their emphasis on the top of the pyramid: the Does level. The Does level requires attention to a robust combination of work-based assessments. It is also critical to recognize that most of all assessment is based on 2 primary activities: asking questions and observing. Exactly how programs and individuals perform these activities varies from assessment method to assessment method.[28] The American Association of Oral and Maxillofacial Surgeons have also published their "Benchmarks in oral and maxillofacial surgery education and training," which also provides a framework with graduated measures that ensure that both the learner and the program faculty understand the basis for the assessment of a resident's progress in various practice domains specific to the specialty.[29]

ADDITIONAL METHODS OF ASSESSING COMPETENCY

A structured OMFS training program must include training in all competencies and not just clinical care. It must identify problems in the learning curve of each resident to allow remediation. The totality of training includes clinical exposure and decision making, preoperative evaluation, postoperative care, the treatment of complications,

independent operating, surgical simulation, and cadaver dissections.[30] Difficult technical operations such as those requiring endoscopy or virtual surgical planning should be candidates for skill development in the skills laboratory, cadaver laboratory, or through surgical simulation, whereby available, before first assisting in the operating room, so as to reduce patient risk due to the steep slope of the resident learning curve.

How then do we improve our ability to develop and assess technical and nontechnical trainee competencies? We must develop and continually improve our surgical curriculum, whereby residents meet certain stages of progress as they pass through the residency. These are commonly referred to as "Milestones" by the ACGME. Each of these stages or milestones is defined by explicit expectations, which can address each of the ACGME/CODA/AAOMS Benchmark competencies. The stages follow the Dreyfus model, which defines professional skills acquisition as occurring in stages whereby one progresses from novice, to beginner, to advanced beginner, to competent/proficient, and eventually some advance to the expert level.[31] The utility of this model for residency training is that progression along these stages can be measured and compared with previously established expectations. Lack of progression will allow early intervention. Assessment of surgical and nontechnical skills is important to recognize problem residents early and apply remediation and document competency before releasing the resident to independent practice. The curriculum should ideally cover all of the ACGME/CODA competencies to produce an OMF surgeon that meets all competencies and not just in the areas of clinical care and medical knowledge. Examples of how those competencies might be evaluated within OMFS residency training programs are outlined in **Table 2**.

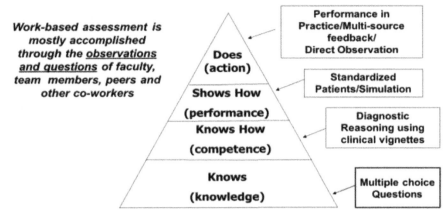

Assessing for the Desired Outcome

Work-based assessment is mostly accomplished through the observations and questions of faculty, team members, peers and other co-workers

Does (action) — Performance in Practice/Multi-source feedback/ Direct Observation

Shows How (performance) — Standardized Patients/Simulation

Knows How (competence) — Diagnostic Reasoning using clinical vignettes

Knows (knowledge) — Multiple choice Questions

Fig. 1. Based on Miller's assessment pyramid,[27] this work-based assessment pyramid demonstrates a framework to assist residency programs in developing their assessment systems. (*From* Accreditation Council for Graduate Medical Education. ACGME Assessment Guidebook. ACGME. Available at: https://www.acgme.org/globalassets/pdfs/milestones/guidebooks/assessmentguidebook.pdf. Accessed January 22, 2022.)

The COVID-19 pandemic also taught us many novel concepts about resident education.[32,33] The capacity to electronically archive education material such as tutorials, lectures, and scientific publications can provide the foundation for "self-directed" learning, learning initiated by the learner, functioning autonomously.[34] However, it should be monitored as the hazard implicit by the incorporation of self-directed learning into the fabric of programmatic resident education is the potential gravitation toward loss of accountability and structure in the absence of interactive teaching.[35] The second element in a process of successful improvement is a concerted embrace of a conceptual conversion of our conference structure from one of a pedagogic ("to lead the child") learning format, dominated by lectures and talks (essentially lectures), to one based on the principles of adult learning[35]: experientially derived learning including the capacity to commit mistakes, problem-oriented rather than teacher-centered, immediate relevance and feedback, ability to apply the information shortly after learning, and participation by the learners in the establishment of their educational goals.[34]

SIMULATION

Transformation of surgical education and concerns for patient safety necessitates novel teaching and assessment methods in training programs.[36] Simulation is an area of educational innovation that maximizes patient safety and allows the trainee to practice all or part of a procedure independently or as part of a team. It has the advantage of a controlled environment and without the common barriers to intraoperative teaching, such as time, attending surgeon teaching approach, and trainee learning style[37] As a surgical specialty, Oral and Maxillofacial Surgery is far behind specialties such as Otorhinolaryngology, Plastic Surgery, General Surgery, Orthopedics and Neurosurgery in the development and application of simulators and their use in residency training programs. Simulation-based learning is a strategy that seeks to create learning outcomes that achieve a level of performance much higher than competence alone. In mastery education, results are uniform, with little variation, although the time to achieve mastery may vary among trainees. Expert performance, particularly in surgery, requires both deliberate and independent practice.[37] The orchestration of an operation involves structured steps (ie, predictable and reproducible) and improvised steps (ie, spontaneous adaptation because of complexity or unexpected findings).[38] Although every operation involves a combination of each of these steps, the more structure that can be applied to a procedure, the greater the likelihood of a predictably excellent surgical outcome.[38] Surgical simulation may be a helpful tool for both the novice and the experienced surgeon who seek to acquire the skills to perform the structured steps of a surgical technique and improvise when necessary. Bell and colleagues observed that methods will have to be developed to allow surgeons to reach a basic level of competence in procedures that they are likely to experience only rarely during residency. Additionally, for even more commonly performed procedures,

Table 2 After AGCME assessment guidebook recommended competencies and assessment methods adapted for OMFS residency training	
Competency	**Competency-Based Assessment Options**
Medical Knowledge	• OMSITE examination • Faculty assessments • Medical pimping
Patient Care and Procedural Skills	• Faculty assessments through the direct observation of the trainee during delivery of care (SIMPL app) • Standardized assessments • Simulation (both technical and nontechnical)
Professionalism	• Informed self-assessment • Multi-source feedback, such as a 360-degree evaluation • Patient experience survey review
Interpersonal and Communication Skills	• Patient-reported feedback and experience surveys • Multi-source feedback, such as a 360-degree evaluation, regarding interprofessional care and communication
Practice-based Learning and Improvement	• Evaluation of knowledge, skills, and attitudes from participation in systemic efforts to improve the quality, safety, or value of OMFS services • Audit and feedback on the medical record • Review of medical errors and patient safety events (M&M) • Evidence-based practice logs
Systems-based Practice	• Feedback from multiple faculty evaluations regarding the ability to practice in a complex health care system *(continued on next page)*

Table 2 *(continued)*	
Competency	**Competency-Based Assessment Options**
	• Multi-source feedback, such as a 360-degree evaluation, especially regarding interprofessional care • Assessment of cost-conscious care

Adapted from Accreditation Council for Graduate Medical Education. ACGME Assessment Guidebook. ACGME. Available at: https://www.acgme.org/globalassets/pdfs/milestones/guidebooks/assessmentguidebook.pdf. Accessed January 22, 2022.

the numbers of repetitions are not robust, stressing the need to determine objectively whether residents are actually achieving basic competency in these operations.[39]

A supportive environment and a curriculum focused on adult learner concepts such as deliberate practice and feedback, along with adjunctive surgical simulation, may be the best way to shorten our resident's learning curve and facilitate skill acquisition with minimal mentoring and maximal patient safety.[40] Simulation on cadaver models has also been shown to be beneficial. However, in many programs, cadaver experience is limited due to myriad factors including cadaver availability and cost. Studies have shown that simulation-based training produces significant increases in both knowledge and skill when compared with more traditional educational methods, including self-directed reading and the use of digital images.[41]

FUTURE CONSIDERATIONS

With regard to the technical competencies we aim to teach our residents, are there a series of commonly performed operations, such as a LeFort I osteotomy, ORIF of a mandibular body fracture, removal of an impacted wisdom tooth, or the placement of a dental implant that would allow a young surgeon to extrapolate those technical skills comfortably to other operations as the specialty evolves? Currently, we teach a smorgasbord of operations based on what is referred into the hospital or walks in through the doors of the emergency room. We hope to achieve more than the minimal number of operations within each CODA category, and if the goal is met, generally deem the graduating resident ready for independent practice as long as they have met the minimum criteria. This one-size-fits-all training may or may not be ideal, although one may make the case that it has served the profession adequately over the last several decades. As we contemplate the future, should we consider modifying our residency programs to focus more on a resident's future practice interests? Most programs do not have the flexibility to accommodate specific tracks within the program. There are elective faculty cases to cover, patients currently in the ED awaiting repair of their facial fracture or drainage of their neck infection, and outpatient clinics to staff. Ideally, we could create more scheduling flexibility, and with this flexibility leverage resources and manpower to improve the focus of preparation of our oral and maxillofacial surgery residents to meet the needs of their future practice goals. With increased flexibility, a more focused and modular approach to support the needs of someone entering a large urban academic practice, which may include greater need for competence in maxillofacial trauma and orthognathic surgery might be designed. Alternatively, one entering private practice may spend more time in the outpatient clinic performing a greater number of dentoalveolar procedures under outpatient anesthesia, dental implant surgery, and bone grafting. In both cases, the minimal number of cases in each CODA category would be reached for each resident, but additional cases would be apportioned based on career trajectory.

We need also to consider the exposure (and subsequent time lost on the OMFS service) that our residents have to other rotations and surgical services. The time for the OMFS trainee to master the skills and techniques that will remain within their long-term scope of practice is limited within every residency program. In many dual degree programs, for instance, the residents serve one or more years as a PGY-1 or PGY-2 general surgery resident. When many of these agreements were put into place several decades ago, most general surgery operations were performed via an open approach. Residents learned proper surgical techniques, became adept at surgical dissection and suturing, and learned many surgical principles that they could then bring back to the oral and maxillofacial surgery service. With the advent of minimally invasive surgery, many OMFS (as well as other surgical subspecialties) are reconsidering and reworking the time spent on general surgery. As an example, would a senior resident's time be better spent participating in laparoscopic colorectal surgery, or acting as a first assist on a bimaxillary orthognathic surgical case? In a named lecture to the Canadian Association of Pediatric Surgeons in 2015, Ronald A. Hirschl[42] noted that "the second major change in residency is the explosion in knowledge, the change in technology, and the movement of cases away from General Surgery, especially complex, open cases. Gastric and duodenal operations are gone for the most part. So are biliary tree and portal vein procedures to GI and IR. Abdominal vascular procedures are now endovascular. Tumor biopsies and venous access are mostly conducted by IR and exploratory laparotomies have been replaced by CT/MRI. Trauma surgery is markedly decreased because of a reduction in penetrating trauma, the advent of CT, and nonoperative options for solid organ injury.[43] Because of the explosion of fellows, many General Surgery residents have become observers during complex cases while on specialty services. Most of the cases are now minimally invasive, thus reducing skill in open operations. Whether open or MIS, it is clear that the exposure of residents to complex operating has been reduced." If this is problematic for general surgery trainees, where does this leave OMFS trainees who are rotating onto General Surgery? In the end, we are training oral and maxillofacial surgeons, not minimally invasive general surgeons. Certainly, there is an overlap between General Surgery and Oral and Maxillofacial Surgery of increasingly independent practice ability, patient responsibility, and some shared motor skills that are fundamental to safe and effective surgical patient care; caring for sick patients in the general surgery service often translate to the patients that we care for on our own service. However, one must consider if the time wouldn't be better spent mastering the problems we treat, the patients we manage, and the operations we perform. Nevertheless, the issue of medical licensure must also be pragmatically weighed in the decision to decrease non-OMFS surgical time in the dual degree program. Modern changes to accreditation and licensure requirements add a significant burden to the graduating dual degree resident hoping to obtain medical licensure. While off-service rotations could potentially add to the resident's skillset in patient management and perioperative care, sufficient core oral and maxillofacial surgery training should not be traded to appease more stringent licensure requirements.[44]

The potential creation of a more tailored experience to improve preparation for the resident's ultimate path in their final year of training is an option. The consideration of which foundational skills should be optimally achieved during OMFS training could be revisited by those who support broad-based training of OMF surgeons. The required prerequisite experiences and skills need to be continually redefined so that the training of our graduates is optimized.

SUMMARY

Traditionally, surgical learning has been based on an apprenticeship model; that is, the long-term observation and assessment of the trainee by his or her seniors over a prolonged period of time.[45] Within academic medical centers and OMFS surgical residency training programs, increased public awareness and expectation of patient safety, work hour restrictions, and mandated increases in faculty oversight have led to decreased resident autonomy and independence. Graduates finishing surgical training with less peri- and intraoperative surgical autonomy may have less confidence and, potentially, less clinical competence, which may affect patient safety, patient outcomes, and career satisfaction. The conventional surgical training model—see one, do one, teach one—lacks the necessary elements to ensure consistent guidance, objective assessment of performance and feedback, and is difficult to justify in terms of patient safety, care, and costs.[46] Response to these changes will require ongoing modification and innovation in both assessment and training methods to ensure that graduates to develop the highest levels of competence and confidence. Each Oral and Maxillofacial Surgery program director must make a decision for the future of our specialty. Do we "stay the course" and spiral downward? Or, do we jettison the outdated modes of our current training programs to become bold and think "out-of-the-box"?[47]

DISCLOSURE

The author has nothing to disclose.

REFERENCES

1. Long DM. Competency-based residency training: The next advance in graduate medical education. Acad Med 2000;75(12):1178–83.
2. Cameron JL. William Stewart Halsted. Our surgical heritage. Ann Surg 1997;225(5):445–58.
3. Hashimoto DA, Sirimanna P, Gomez ED, et al. Deliberate practice enhances quality of laparoscopic surgical performance in a randomized controlled trial: from arrested development to expert performance. Surg Endosc 2015;29(11):3154–62.
4. Gawande AA, Thomas EJ, Zinner MJ, et al. The incidence and nature of surgical adverse events in Colorado and Utah in 1992. Surg 1999;126(1):66–75.
5. Leape LL, Brennan TA, Laird N, et al. The nature of adverse events in hospitalized patients. Results of the Harvard Medical Practice Study II. N Engl J Med 1991;324(6):377–84.
6. Thomas EJ, Studdert DM, Newhouse JP, et al. Costs of medical injuries in Utah and Colorado. Inquiry Fall 1999;36(3):255–64.
7. Balasundaram I, Aggarwal R, Darzi LA. Development of a training curriculum for microsurgery. Br J Oral Maxillofac Surg 2010;48(8):598–606.
8. Americal Dental Association Commission on Dental Accreditation. Accreditation standards for advanced dental education programs in oral and maxillofacial surgery. Available at: https://coda.ada.org/~/media/CODA/Files/oms.pdf?la=en. Accessed December 22, 2021.
9. Nygaard R, Daly S, Camp J. General surgery resident case logs: Do they accurately reflect resident experience? J Surg Educ 2015;72:e178–83.
10. American Board of Oral and Maxillofacial Surgery. OMSITE. Available at: https://www.aboms.org/omsite. Accessed January 2, 2022.
11. Carlson ER. Medical pimping versus the Socratic method of teaching. J Oral Maxillofac Surg 2017;75(1):3–5.
12. Jaffer A, Bednarz B, Challacombe B, et al. The assessment of surgical competency in the UK. Int J Surg 2009;7(1):12–5.
13. Paisley AM, Baldwin PJ, Paterson-Brown S. Validity of surgical simulation for the assessment of operative skill. Br J Surg 2001;88(11):1525–32.
14. Bridgewater B, Grayson AD, Jackson M, et al. Surgeon specific mortality in adult cardiac surgery: comparison between crude and risk stratified data. Br Med J 2003;327(7405):13–7.
15. Binenbaum G, Musick DW, Ross HM. The development of physician confidence during surgical and medical internship. Am J Surg 2007;193(1):79–85.
16. Lewis FR, Klingensmith ME. Issues in general surgery residency training—2012. Ann Surg 2012;256(4):553–9.
17. Tannyhill RJ, Baron M, Troulis MJ. Do graduating oral-maxillofacial surgery residents feel confident in practicing the full scope of the specialty? J Oral Maxillofac Surg 2021;79(2):286–94.
18. Coleman JJ, Esposito TJ, Rozycki GS, et al. Early subspecialization and perceived competence in surgical training: Are residents ready? J Am Coll Surg 2013;216(4):764–71.
19. Stulberg JJ, Huang R, Kreutzer L, et al. Association between surgeon technical skills and patient outcomes. JAMA Surg 2020;155(10):960–8.
20. Safavi A, Lai S, Butterworth S, et al. Does operative experience during residency correlate with reported competency of recent general surgery graduates? Can J Surg 2012;55(4):S171–7.
21. Healey P, Samanta J. When does the 'learning curve' of innovative interventions become questionable practice? Eur J Vasc Endovasc Surg 2008;36(3):253–7.

22. McQueen S, McKinnon V, VanderBeek L, et al. Video-based assessment in surgical education: a scoping review. J Surg Educ 2019;76(6): 1645–54.

23. George BC, Teitelbaum EN, Meyerson SL, et al. Reliability, validity, and feasibility of the Zwisch scale for the assessment of intraoperative performance. J Surg Educ 2014;71(6):e90–6.

24. Kaban LB, Cappetta A, George BC, et al. Evaluation of oral and maxillofacial surgery residents' operative skills: Feasibility and engagement study using SIMPL software for a mobile phone. J Oral Maxillofac Surg 2017;75(10):2041–7.

25. Bohnen JD, George BC, Williams RG, et al. The Feasibility of Real-Time Intraoperative Performance Assessment With SIMPL (System for Improving and Measuring Procedural Learning): Early Experience From a Multi-institutional Trial. J Surg Educ 2016;73(6):e118–30.

26. Sonnadara R, McQueen S, Mironova P, et al. Reflections on current methods for evaluating skills during joint replacement surgery: a scoping review. Bone Joint J 2013;95-B(11):1445–9.

27. Miller GE. The assessment of clinical skills/competence/performance. Acad Med 1990;65(9):S63–7.

28. Accreditation Council for Graduate Medical Education. ACGME assessment guidebook. ACGME. Available at: https://www.acgme.org/globalassets/pdfs/milestones/guidebooks/assessmentguidebook.pdf. Accessed January 22, 2022.

29. American Association of Oral and Maxillofacial Surgeons. Benchmarks in oral and maxillofacial surgery education and training. Available at: https://www.aaoms.org/docs/education_research/edu_training/oms_benchmarks.pdf. Accessed Dec 24, 2021.

30. Hashem AM, Waltzman JT, D'Souza GF, et al. Resident and program director perceptions of aesthetic training in plastic surgery residency: An update. Aesth Surg J 2017;37(7):837–46.

31. Mukhtar M, Gunderman RB. The sixth stage: mastery. Acad Radiol 2017;24(12):1621–3.

32. Mohan AT, Vyas KS, Asaad M, et al. Plastic surgery lockdown learning during coronavirus disease 2019: are adaptations in education here to stay? Plas Reconstr Surg Glob Open 2020;8(7):e3064.

33. Moe J, Brookes C, Dyalram D, et al. Resident education in the time of a global pandemic: development of the collaborative OMS virtual interinstitutional didactic (COVID) program. J Oral Maxillofac Surg 2020;78(8):1224–6.

34. Luce EA. Graduate plastic surgery education and seventy-five years of plastic and reconstructive surgery. Plast Reconstr Surg 2021;48(6):1429–35.

35. Luce EA. The future of plastic surgery resident education. Plas Reconstruc Surg 2016;137(3):1063–70.

36. Nathwani JN, Fiers RM, Ray RD, et al. Relationship between technical errors and decision-making skills in the junior resident. J Surg Educ 2016;73(6): e84–90.

37. Tannyhill RJ, Jensen OT. Computer simulation training for mandibular all-on-four/all-on-three surgery. Oral Maxillofacial Surg Clin N Am 2019;31(3): 505–11.

38. Dearani JA, Gold M, Leibovich BC, et al. The role of imaging, deliberate practice, structure, and improvisation in approaching surgical perfection. J Thorac Cardiovasc Surg 2017;154(4):1329–36.

39. Bell RH Jr, Biester TW, Tabuenca A, et al. Operative experience of residents in US general surgery programs: A gap between expectation and experience. Ann Surg 2009;249.

40. Tannyhill RJ, Jensen OT. Computer simulation and maxillary all-on-four surgery. Oral Maxillofac Surg Clin North Am 2019;31:497–504.

41. O'Neill R, Raj S, Davis MJ, et al. Aesthetic training in plastic surgery residency. Plas Reconstruc Surg Glob Open 2020;8(7):e2895.

42. Hirschl RB. The making of a surgeon: 10,000 hours? J Pediatr Surg 2015;50(5):699–706.

43. Klingensmith ME, Lewis FR. General surgery residency training issues. Adv Surg 2013;47(1): 251–70. d.

44. Ganjawalla KP, Jazayeri HE, Moe JS, et al. Dual degree training: Balancing clinical aptitude and medical licensure requirements. J Oral Maxillofac Surg 2021;79(10):1988–90.

45. Lee AG, Beaver HA, Greenlee E, et al. Teaching and assessing systems-based competency in ophthalmology residency training programs. Surv Ophthalmol 2007;52:680–9.

46. Tay C, Khajuria A, Gupte C. Simulation training: A systematic review of simulation in arthroscopy and proposal of a new competency-based training framework. Int J Surg 2014;12(6):626–33.

47. Rohrich RJ. The making of a plastic surgeon: Present and future. Plas Reconstruc Surg 2021; 148(5S):25S–6S.

Changing Dynamics of Accreditation in Oral and Maxillofacial Surgery

Sruthi Satishchandran, DMD[a],*, Catherine Horan, PhD[b],
Steven Roser, DMD, MD, FACS, FRCSEd[c]

KEYWORDS

- Accreditation • Commission on Dental Accreditation • (CODA)
- The accreditation Council for Graduate Medical Education (ACGME) • Competency-based training

KEY POINTS

- The Commission on Dental Accreditation has made and continues to make changes to support oral and maxillofacial surgery programs.
- Changes in the public's awareness of challenges in the current health care delivery have led to their expectations that surgeons will be leaders in making changes in the system. To do this training programs need to make changes that better the next generation of surgeons.
- Competency-based education programs will be built on platforms of standard curriculum, valid outcome assessment of trainees while in the program and at the end of the program.
- These changes will require changes in the accreditation system from one that focuses on assurance of compliance with standards to include assisting programs with outcome.
- The next step in the evolution of accreditation for oral and maxillofacial surgery training programs and their accreditation will require agreement by all the stakeholders.

INTRODUCTION

Accreditation is a review process by which a designated accrediting organization determines whether educational programs, health care facilities, and other programs meet the standards of quality. Once achieved, the accreditation is renewed periodically to ensure that the quality is maintained. Accreditation, as a requirement, may vary for different countries. In the United States, programs are accredited by 1 of the 60 recognized accreditation organizations. Accrediting organizations that are approved for this process are reviewed by the Council for Higher Education (CHEA) or the United States Department of Education (USDE). The CHEA database contains information about more than 8000 institutions and 44,000 programs in the United States. The Commission of Dental Accreditation (CODA) is one of the recognized accreditation organizations in the CHEA database. The process of dental educational program accreditation has a long history that continues to change and develop new methodology.

BACKGROUND

CODA is the current organization that assesses compliance with the published standards to monitor and control the continuous quality of dental education programs. From 1938 to 1974 the American Dental Association's Council on Dental Education was the recognized agency for accreditation for dental education programs. In

---

[a] Oral and Maxillofacial Surgery Resident-in-Training, Division of Oral and Maxillofacial Surgery, Department of Surgery, Emory University School of Medicine, Atlanta, GA, USA; [b] Retired Consultant for the Commission on Dental Accreditation; [c] DeLos Hill Chair and Professor of Surgery and Chief of Division of Oral and Maxillofacial Surgery, Emory University School of Medicine, 1365 Clifton RoadSuite B2300, Atlanta, GA 30322, USA
* Corresponding author.
E-mail address: sruthi.satishchandran@emory.edu

Oral Maxillofacial Surg Clin N Am 34 (2022) 515–519
https://doi.org/10.1016/j.coms.2022.03.003
1042-3699/22/© 2022 Elsevier Inc. All rights reserved.

1972, CODA was formed, and since 1975 it has been nationally recognized by the USDA and CHEA as the sole organization that accredits all dental education programs, including dental schools, advanced dental education programs, and allied dental education programs in the United States.

The foundation of CODA's accreditation process is the self-study and the binary form of site visit and Education review committee/Commission review.[1] The primary role of the Site Visit Team is to gather and evaluate data submitted in the self-study by the institution or program. Members of the dental school site visit team includes those with expertise in biomedical science, clinical oral health care, administration, and finance. The site visitors for the advanced dental education programs are specialty specific. The site visitors are volunteers except when CODA staff accompany dental school site visit teams. Programs perform a self-assessment through the Self-Study process. To assess compliance, the site visitors review the self-study materials and visit the programs during which they interview faculty and trainees, tour the facilities, review the curriculum, and discuss any recommendations with the program and sponsoring institution leadership. The Site Visitors Evaluation Report (SEVR) is sent to CODA. The report is reviewed by CODA administration staff and sent back to the program leadership for comment. Any program comments are included with the SEVR and the Self-Study.[2] The combined report is reviewed by the CODA School or Specialty Education Review Committee. The program has the opportunity to appear before the Education Review Committee to discuss the SEVR. The Education Review Committee's recommendations are then forwarded to the Commission Board for final action. Final actions include accreditation without reporting, accreditation with reporting, and intent to withdraw accreditation.[2] The intent of this process is to assist the programs to comply with the standards.

The Accreditation Council for Graduate Medical Education (ACGME) is a private not-for-profit institution that sets standards for United States medical education residencies and fellowships. The ACGME was founded in 1981 by the American Board of Medical Specialties, American Hospital Association, American Medical Association, and the Association on Medical Colleges.

The ACGME accreditation process includes a program Self-Study in which programs self-report strengths and areas of improvement. There is also an accreditation process in which an institution that sponsors postgraduate medical education programs completes a self-study that analyzes the GME performance at that specific institution and assures competence with institutional standards.[3] The site visits for ACGME programs are typically performed by Accreditation Field Representatives who are employed by the ACGME, except in special circumstances for specialty programs in which the site visitors may be specialty specific. Similar to CODA site visitors, the ACGME site visitors are not the decision-makers, rather they collect and aggregate relevant data, which they compile into a narrative known that the Site Visit Report. Subsequently, this report is used by the ACGME Review and Recognition Committees to make accreditation or recommendation decisions.[3]

In 1999, the ACGME introduced competency-based training as a goal for all postgraduate medical education programs. Residents were expected to demonstrate competency in 6 domains, including patient care, medical knowledge, interpersonal communication skills, professionalism, practice-based learning and improvement, and systems-based practice. Within these domains, with input from the specialties, the Specialty Milestones were developed that are used to assess resident progress throughout the program and at the final evaluation.[4]

Competency-based educational models are present in many fields and are often called competency-based education and training (CBET).[4] Within the realm of medicine this term became known as "CBME." As Sullivan notes "In a traditional educational system, the unit of progression is time- and teacher-centered. In a CBET system, the unit of progression is mastery of specific knowledge and skills and is learner-centered".[5]

CBET had much of its origins linked to the teacher education reform movement of the 1960s.[6] In 1978, McGaghie and his colleagues promoted competency-based models for medical education as part of a report to the World Health Organization.[7] In that report, the investigators described the goal of CBME as follows: "The intended output of a competency-based program is a health professional who can practice medicine at a defined level of proficiency, in accord with local conditions, to meet local needs."[8,9]

In 2002, Carraccio described a 4-step process for implementing CBME: (1) identification of the competencies (in the United States the 6 ACGME Core Competencies); (2) determination of competency components and performance levels (eg, benchmarks and milestones); (3) competency assessment; and (4) overall evaluation of the process.[10]

CBME allows learners to progress through an educational program at different rates. This results in the fast learners making transitions in their training earlier. Others, who require more time to gain the knowledge and skills necessary for their medical career, are able to be given that time within the program. A second unique feature of CBME is the increased emphasis on ongoing assessment, allowing faculty to determine the developmental progress of the learner and the learner to receive frequent feedback, coaching, and adjustments to their learning plans.[11–13]

TOOLS USED FOR ORAL AND MAXILLOFACIAL SURGERY ACCREDITATION

1. Accreditation Standards for Advanced Dental Education Programs in Oral and Maxillofacial Surgery
2. Annual Survey
3. Self-Study document

The Oral and Maxillofacial Surgery Accreditation Process

The Commission on Dental Accreditation's accreditation process for advanced dental education programs is a standardized and accepted method of evaluation that, at the minimum, reassures society and the profession that there is compliance by the programs with published standards. With all accreditation processes, there is a front and a back end. The front end is a Self-Study in which policies and procedures are evaluated by the institution or program. The back end of the accreditation process is a Site Visit, with a report, to confirm what is reported in the Self-Study and a review of both by the accrediting body. OMS is on a 5-year cycle for accreditation. Dental schools and the other advanced dental education programs are on a 7-year cycle.

CODA-accredited fellowships are unique to the specialties of OMS and Orthodontics. The OMS fellowship accreditation process is similar to the OMS residency accreditation process. There are 12 accredited OMS fellowship programs as of February 2022.

Annual Survey

The Annual Survey collects important data for the on-going quality assessment of the programs under the purview of CODA. Common standards, which are put into place by CODA, are the same for all advanced dental education programs.[2,3] The specialties' standards and changes in standards are proposed by the specialty to CODA. They are subject to public review and a vote by the accrediting body before implementing them. Information on Program Surveys can be accessed at the following: https://coda.ada.org/en/find-a-program/program-surveys. In addition to providing CODA the opportunity to provide ongoing reviews of the advanced dental education program compliance with the standards, the annual survey permits CODA to aggregate 5-year data for the site visits.[3]

DISCUSSION
The Movement of CODA Toward an Independent Accrediting Agency

Some activities within CODA involve independent commission committees that use commission strategies to progress major action items at each meeting. One action item that was progressed was a discussion of areas of improvement to lead to CODA becoming an independent accreditation agency.

Accreditation Changes During the COVID-19 Pandemic

On March 13, 2020, a national emergency was declared due to the COVID 19 pandemic. Because of the significant impact on travel, CODA determined the use of alternate site visits to be appropriate. This involved virtual or hybrid site visit methods to maintain CODA's commitment to conduct site visits to currently accredited US dental education programs or US programs applying for accreditation. The hybrid site visit would involve at least 1 on-site consultant, whereas in the virtual alternative all site visitors can be remote. Historically CODA had not used virtual site visits.[14]

Hybrid site visits were organized to include all components of the site visit process. With both the virtual and on-site review of the program by at least one commission member, all areas of assessment would be fulfilled. The Commission views the hybrid site visit as equivalent to an on-site visit, with no subsequent visit required. Following the virtual (and on-site visit within 18 months) or hybrid site visit, the program's next reaccreditation on-site visit will be scheduled in 5 years following the date of the virtual or hybrid site visit.[14]

In addition, during the COVID 19 pandemic, there was a *temporary flexibility guidance* given on select Accreditation Standards. For the Class of 2021, there was a modification of curriculum content, program-dictate requirements, and CODA's quantitative numbers–based requirements. Although there were no changes made to the minimum program length and rotation lengths, the use of alternate knowledge-based education methods was acceptable.[14,15] Distanced learning via conferencing technology, simulations, and web-based resources were permissible in lieu of in-person formal instruction, in-person literature reviews, and multidisciplinary grand rounds. Discretion was given to the program director to ensure competence of its graduated residents.[15]

Institutional Review Committee as Another Measure of Evaluation

A unique characteristic of ACGME is the separate accreditation of the Sponsoring Institution that supports one or more ACGME-accredited residency or fellowship programs. A governing body (single person or group) has responsibility for graduate medical education (GME) within the Sponsoring Institution, and there is an institutional official (DIO) at the Sponsoring Institution who is accountable to the ACGME and the Sponsoring Institution.[3] A local GME committee is required by the ACGME to ensure the accredited programs are complying with ACGME institutional, common, and specialty-/subspecialty-specific program requirements. The GME committee must demonstrate effective oversight of the Sponsoring Institution's accreditation through an Annual Institutional Review and institutional site visits.[3]

Advanced dental education programs sponsored by schools of dentistry are in part supported by the school. The OMS residency training programs that are sponsored by dental schools have a strong presence in hospital need to comply with both hospital and dental school institutional policies regarding graduate medical education. These programs and the OMS programs sponsored by medical schools or hospitals find themselves in a unique situation living in an ACGME environment and being accredited by CODA; this can provide challenges to accessing the resources for their training programs to meet the changes in health care delivery and expectations for a specialty of surgery.

SUMMARY

CODA is a dynamic agency that has made significant changes to OMS accreditation standards since its inauguration, best exemplified by the "temporary guidance" made during the state of emergency during the COVID-19 pandemic. CODA was able to addend standards for compliance and work with program directors to ensure the competence of the graduates. Accreditation is defined by CODA as the process that ensures residents, the dental profession, specialty boards, and the public that accredited training programs are in compliance with published standards (Accreditation Standards for Advanced Dental Education Programs In Oral

and Maxillofacial Surgery, Commission on Dental Accreditation June 2021). This process is a combined effort between our professions (AAOMS), and the professional evaluators (CODA). It provides a consistent and equitable process to assure compliance with the published standards for oral and maxillofacial training programs. CODA and our profession are continuously modifying the standards to meet the changing demands of oral and maxillofacial surgery postgraduate training. Increasing public awareness of health care delivery has led to the expectation by the public that surgeons are leaders in patient care delivery, are well versed in the use of systems needed to improve health care delivery including informational technology, understand the disparities in health care, and are culturally sensitive and cost conscious in addition to being clinically competent. Changes are necessary to the education and training programs and the accreditation system to meet these expectations. Accreditation systems need to place more focus on outcome and assessing the residents' progress during training at the end of training and beyond. To do this there could include a reduction in proscriptive standards, establishing a set of core standards and an increase in the role of the program and the program's institution in the design of the education and training. To do this CODA will need to add to its predominately compliance assurance role to include assisting the programs to provide effective high-quality education in a safe learning environment. The incentive to strive for excellence will come from the programs, the program's sponsoring institution, as well as the program's compliance with their published specialty standards.

This process will only work if there is trust between the accrediting body, the sponsoring institution, and its programs. Support for the ongoing trust is maintained by the ACGME by the postgraduate medical programs and their residents and faculty continuously reporting outcome data directly to the ACGME. These data include surgical and anesthesia logs, duty hours, and annual surveys of the residents and the faculty addressing the educational program, the learning environment and their satisfaction with it. This process allows the ACGME to provide accountability of the program and the sponsoring institutions' educational programs' effectiveness to society and the profession. Similarly, CODA could function as an accrediting body for institutions sponsoring an oral and maxillofacial surgery training program using the continuous reporting of outcome data from the programs directly to CODA to provide accountability.

Oral and maxillofacial surgery is currently in a unique position to undertake the changes in the training programs and their accreditation which are being called for by the public, the profession the faculty and the trainees. The introduction of a national curriculum, The SCORE Curriculum Outline for Oral and Maxillofacial Surgery, is a keystone for making the changes. On the platform provided by a standard curriculum for all OMS training programs, the benchmarks that have been already developed by our specialty can be better implemented, assessed, modified, and validated. Validated benchmarks are a second keystone and with the standard curriculum will be the platform for establishing a competency-based curriculum that will provide effective assessment of the progress of the resident in the training program and achievement of the final benchmarks will provide assurance to society and the profession that the trainee meets the high-quality standards set by the profession for an independent practitioner. The American Board of Oral and Maxillofacial Surgery in turn should have a better platform to provide an effective maintenance of certification program.

These changes in the accreditation process for oral and maxillofacial surgery programs can provide the programs with the flexibility to better tailor the program for the individual trainee. Competency-based training allows for new opportunities for the fast learners and opportunities for remediation for those who require more time and guidance with the core program. There is some urgency to undertaking the process necessary to make these changes. The changes need to be well thought out. Input must come from all the stakeholders. Thought leaders and resources are available, as medical postgraduate training programs are facing the same challenges. The time to begin is now.

DISCLOSURE

The authors have nothing to disclose.

REFERENCE

1. Commission on dental accreditation evaluation and operational policies and procedures manual. Available at: https://anthc.org/wp-content/uploads/2020/02/EOPP-2019.pdf. Accessed Feb 20, 2022.

2. Accreditation Standards for Advanced Dental Education Programs in Oral and Maxillofacial Surgery. 2021. Available at: https://coda.ada.org/~/media/CODA/Files/oms.pdf?la=en. Accessed Feb 19,2022.

3. ACGME Common Program Requirements. 2019. Available at: https://www.acgme.org/Portals/0/ PFAssets/ProgramRequirements/CPRResidency 2019.pdf. Accessed Feb 26, 2022.

4. Achike Francis I, Lakhan SE, Yakub M. Competency-based Medical Education: Philosophy, What, How, Why, and the Challenges Therein. J Med Educ 2019;23(1):1–13.

5. Sullivan, Rick L. The competency-based approach to training. Strategy paper No 1. Baltimore, Maryland: JHPIEGO Corporation; 1995.

6. Elam Stanley. Performance-based teacher education: what is the state of the art? Washington: American Association of Colleges for Teacher Education; 1971. p. 1–36.

7. McGaghie WC, Lipson L. Competency-based curriculum development in medical education: an introduction. Public health papers, 68. Geneva: World Health Organization; 1978.

8. Whitcomb ME. Transforming medical education. Acad Med 2016;91(5):618–20.

9. VanMelle E Van, Frank JR, Holmboe ES, et al. A core components framework for evaluating implementation of competency-based medical education programs. Acad Med 2019;94(7):1002–9.

10. Carraccio C, Wolfsthal SD, Englander R, et al. Shifting paradigms: from flexner to competencies. Acad Med 2002;77(5):361–7. https://doi.org/10.1097/00001888-200205000-00003.

11. Englander R, Frank JR, Carraccio C, et al. Toward a shared language for competency-based medical education. Med Teach 2017;39(6):582–7.

12. Holmboe ES, Sherbino J, Long DM, et al. The role of assessing in competency-based medical education. Med Teach 2010;32:676–82.

13. Ferguson PC, Caverzagie KJ, Nousiainen MT, et al. Changing the Culture of Medical Training: An Important Step toward the Implementation of Competency-Based Medical Education. Med Teach 2017;39(6):599–602. https://doi.org/10.1080/0142159x.2017.1315079.

14. Guidance document: temporary flexibility in accreditation standards to address interruption of education reporting requirements resulting from COVID-19 for the class of 2021. September/October Available at: https://coda.ada.org/~/media/CODA/Files/COVID_Guidelines_InterruptionofEducation_Classof2021.pdf?la=en2020. Accessed February 20, 2022.

15. CODA Special Closed Meeting October 13, 2020 - Unofficial Report of Major Actions. 2020. Available at: https://coda.ada.org/~/media/CODA/Files/CODA_Alert_Special_Closed_Meeting.pdf?la=en. Accessed Feb 20, 2022.

Certification by the American Board of Oral and Maxillofacial Surgery
Residency to Retirement

Vincent J. Perciaccante, DDS[a,b,]*, Larry L. Cunningham Jr, DDS, MD[c]

KEYWORDS

• Board certification • Certification maintenance • OMSITE • QE • OCE

KEY POINTS

- The continuum of the board certification process in oral and maxillofacial surgery begins in residency. The process continues through the examination process and onward with Certification Maintenance and lifelong learning.
- The staff, directors, and Examination Committee volunteers put all testing material through a rigorous process for construction, calibration, and psychometric analysis, to provide a fair and valid examination process.
- The examinations by the American Board of Oral and Maxillofacial Surgery, have and will continue to, evolve over time to remain contemporary within the field and the educational landscape.

INTRODUCTION

Certification by the American Board of Oral and Maxillofacial Surgery (ABOMS) is considered by many to be the crowning achievement of an oral and maxillofacial surgeon's professional education. Obtaining board certification, and continuing to be certified, can be considered a continuum. The process of certification begins in residency and continues until the surgeon retires from surgical practice. Board certification provides personal satisfaction of achievement, evidence to the public that the surgeon strives to apply the highest levels of care in their practice, and that they subscribe to the ABOMS Canons of Ethical Conduct.[1]

Like many high-functioning boards, the ABOMS will, at regular intervals, undergo long-range planning and strategic planning. At the time of this writing, the most recent strategic planning meeting was in December 2021. At that time the Directors and staff of the ABOMS revised the board's Mission and Vision statements.

Mission: The ABOMS ensures that diplomates meet our standards of training, education, and professionalism through our certification process. As the certifying body in oral and maxillofacial surgery, the ABOMS provides contemporary and innovative programs that promote optimal care and service to the public.

Vision: To be the recognized leader in board certification for oral and maxillofacial surgery and related disciplines.

BRIEF HISTORY

The ABOMS was first incorporated in Illinois as The American Board of Oral Surgery on March 19, 1946.[2] This incorporation followed over a

[a] Division of Oral and Maxillofacial Surgery, Emory University School of Medicine, Atlanta, GA, USA; [b] Private Practice, South Oral and Maxillofacial Surgery, 406 Stevens Entry, Peachtree City, GA 30269, USA; [c] Department of Oral and Maxillofacial Surgery, University of Pittsburgh School of Dental Medicine, Salk Hall; UPitt SDM, 3501 Terrace Street; Suite 427, Pittsburgh, PA 15213, USA
* Corresponding author. South Oral and Maxillofacial Surgery, 406 Stevens Entry, Peachtree City, GA 30269.
E-mail address: vpercia@emory.edu
Twitter: @llcunn2 (L.L.C.)

Oral Maxillofacial Surg Clin N Am 34 (2022) 521–528
https://doi.org/10.1016/j.coms.2022.03.011

decade of discussion and collaboration on the topic within the American Society of Oral Surgeons. The formation was approved on April 9, 1946, by the American Dental Association's Council on Dental Education (now replaced by the National Commission on Recognition of Dental Specialties and Certifying Boards), and by the authority of the American Dental Association (ADA) House of Delegates. The final Articles of Incorporation were duly registered in November of 1946. Dr Howard C. Miller served as the first president of the Board from 1946 to 1950. The first examination was given at the Stevens Hotel, in Chicago, February 14 to 15, 1947. In 1978 the board adopted the current designation, the American Board of Oral and Maxillofacial Surgery, following the lead of the American Association of Oral and Maxillofacial Surgeons (AAOMS).

Structure of the American Board of Oral and Maxillofacial Surgery

The ABOMS Board of Directors (BOD) consists of 8 surgeons who are selected from the Examination Committee. The 8-year term is progressive; Directors serve in a section consultant role for 4 years, followed by a year as secretary/treasurer, vice president and Oral Certifying Examination (OCE) chair, president of the board, and finally immediate past-president.

The election process begins with self-nominations from the Examination Committee. Candidates must have served 3 of the last 5 years as an examiner for the OCE. All self-nominations are accompanied by 2 letters of recommendation from current committee members and a statement of interest from the candidate. Applications are reviewed by the current BOD, and then a standardized interview process is carried out. Following the interviews, the BOD presents a slate of nominees to the current Examination Committee, who vote and select 3 names to be forwarded to the AAOMS Board of Trustees and on to a vote by the AAOMS House of Delegates at the AAOMS Annual Meeting. The final candidate is installed as a Director by a vote of the current BOD.

As with many nonprofit boards, the real work is done by dedicated staff members. The ABOMS is proud of its staff members; an Executive Vice President, a vice president for credentialing programs and operations, a director of certification programs services and communications services, a manager of certification services and communications, a manager of programs and operations, 2 examination services coordinators, and an administrative assistant.

ABOMS Administration
Erin Killeen, Executive Vice President
Adrianna Lagunas, Vice President, Credentialing Programs and Operations
Courtney Walsh, Director, Certification Programs Services and Communication Services
Katie Moore, Manager, Certification Services and Communications
Raquel Kalfus, Manager, Program and Operations
Linh Vo, Examination Services Coordinator
Gwyneth Helm, Examination Services Coordinator
Angel Ortiz, Administrative Assistant

EXAMINATIONS

The ABOMS currently administers 3 examinations on an annual basis and 2 examinations on a biennial basis.

Oral and Maxillofacial Surgery In-service Training Examination

The Oral and Maxillofacial Surgery In-service Training Examination (OMSITE) is a 250-question computer-based examination designed to measure the knowledge base and competencies of residents in the field of oral and maxillofacial surgery. The OMSITE is typically administered in computer-testing centers in February of each year to residents in accredited oral and maxillofacial surgery training programs in the United States and Canada. The OMSITE covers 10 subject areas designed to reflect the knowledge and skills of participating residents. This examination is designed to assist residents in assessing their own fund of knowledge, and it provides an objective assessment to program directors as they guide residents through the didactic curriculum.

Qualifying Examination

The Qualifying Examination (QE) is a computer-based examination designed to test knowledge in the central principles of the oral and maxillofacial surgery specialty. The first step in the ABOMS board certification process, this examination contains 300-350 questions covering 10 subject areas. The QE is administered at computer-testing centers in January each year to practicing oral and maxillofacial surgeons. In 2021 the ABOMS began offering a Fast-Track for senior residents. With approval from their program director, those residents in their last year of training may take the QE before graduating from their oral and maxillofacial surgery program. Successful completion of the QE makes a candidate eligible to apply for the OCE.

Oral Certifying Examination

The OCE is an oral examination designed to test a candidate's knowledge, judgment, and critical thinking in the field of oral and maxillofacial surgery. The examination is administered in a standardized testing center in January-February each year. Leading up to the 2019 administration, the examination underwent the first major restructuring in many years, resulting in the current 3-section format. This restructuring was based on the strategic plan of the ABOMS, years of examiner and examinee comments, Commision on Dental Accreditation (CODA) standards for residency training, current and potential future testing sites, psychometric input in multiple aspects/facets of the examination, Director content weighting/averaging, and observation of other specialty certification processes. The second step in the ABOMS board certification process, the examination consists of these 3 sections, each with four 12-minute cases, for a total of 144 minutes. Successful completion of the OCE results in being formally recognized as a Diplomate of ABOMS.

Certificates of Added Qualifications

The Board offers 2 Certificates of Added Qualifications (CAQ) for diplomates who demonstrate education, training, and experience in specialized areas, and who conduct a practice with emphasis on, and commitment to, these focused surgical disciplines. The 2 CAQs offered by ABOMS are Head and Neck Oncologic and Reconstructive Surgery and Pediatric Craniomaxillofacial Surgery (Cleft and Craniofacial). Fellowship-trained individuals may apply to take the CAQ after submitting a case list that meets a minimum criterion in number of cases and case complexity. These 100-question examinations are computer based and are typically administered in November of even-numbered years.

The CAQ examinations were developed in response to a desire of diplomates who had obtained fellowship-level education and training to inform the public and professional colleagues that an oral and maxillofacial surgeon who holds this certification is qualified to practice within this focused specialty area. The creation of the CAQ does not imply exclusion of other practitioners. However, after considering contemporary professional landscape with regard to "shared expertise"

among several competing surgical specialties, the Board thought that offering CAQs provided further evidence of qualification of diplomates to focus practices on subspecialty disciplines.

The ABOMS continuously monitors and provides input toward the accreditation standards for training in oral and maxillofacial surgery. Representatives for the ABOMS sit on the Commission on Dental Accreditation's Residency Review Committee as well as the American Association of Oral and Maxillofacial Surgery's Committee on Education and Training.

Approximately every 5 years the American Board of Oral and Maxillofacial Surgery undertakes a comprehensive review of the contemporary practice of oral and maxillofacial surgeons by administering a survey of practice analysis. The most recent practice analysis enlisted 17 subject matter experts for a task force to identify knowledge and skill statements for use in the survey. The task force then provided guidelines for item development.

In 2021, surveys were sent to 2200 diplomates who fit the following criteria:

- Diplomates less than 2 year out from training
- Mid-career Diplomates (5–10 years from training)
- Diplomates who identify as hospital-affiliated practices.

This was an online survey, taking approximately 30 minutes to complete. There were 475 responses received and used to validate the tasks and knowledge that are important to the work performed by oral and maxillofacial surgery professionals. These interactions guide the creation, maintenance, and updating of the blueprints for each examination and resulted in updates to the QE item bank in 2021. A similar process was used for the significant changes to the OCE that occurred in 2019.

Blueprints

Each examination starts with a "blueprint," or an outline that gives an aspirational number of items from each domain and topic area. Blueprints are created with the help of practice and educational surveys, attention to accreditation requirements, and with knowledge of contemporary practice of oral and maxillofacial surgery (**Boxes 1–4**).

EXAMINATION COMMITTEE LEADERSHIP STRUCTURE

The current OCE is broken up into 3 Surgery sections and a section of Certification Maintenance,

Box 1
Oral and maxillofacial surgery in-service training examination blueprint

I. Medical assessment and management of the surgical patient

  A. Cardiovascular

  B. Respiratory

  C. Musculoskeletal and nervous system

  D. Endocrine, Gastrointestinal, Genitourinary, metabolic

II. Anesthesia and pain control

  A. Local anesthesia

  B. Deep sedation/general anesthesia

  C. Advanced Cardiac Life Support

  D. Perioperative pain control

  E. Pediatric anesthesia/Pediatric Advanced Life Support

III. Dentoalveolar

  A. Erupted/unerupted teeth

  B. Dentoalveolar injuries

  C. Infections

  D. Soft tissue procedures

IV. Trauma

  A. Evaluation of the patients with trauma /Advanced Trauma Life Support

  B. Mandibular injuries

  C. Mid/upper facial injuries

  D. Soft tissue injuries

V. Orthognathic/cleft/Obstructive Sleep Apnea

  A. Mandibular deformities

  B. Maxillary deformities

  C. Cleft lip and palate

  D. Craniofacial syndromes

  E. Obstructive sleep apnea

VI. Cosmetic

  A. Nasal

  B. Periorbital

  C. Skeletal contour alteration

  D. Soft tissue procedures

VII. Temporomandibular disorders/facial pain

  A. Muscular disorders

  B. Internal derangements

  C. Degenerative joint disease

  D. Joint and disk reconstruction

  E. Facial pain

VIII. Pathology

  A. Benign lesions of hard tissue

  B. Benign lesions of soft tissue

  C. Mucocutaneous dermatopathology

  D. Salivary gland pathology

  E. Malignant lesions of hard tissue

  F. Malignant lesions of soft tissue

IX. Reconstruction

  A. Nonvascularized hard tissue grafts

  B. Nonvascularized soft tissue grafts

  C. Vascularized grafts

  D. Pedicle flap

X. Implants

  A. Biology and treatment planning

  B. Prosthetic considerations

  C. Hard tissue adjunctive measures/ distraction osteogenesis

  D. Soft tissue adjunctive measures

  E. Complications

each section having the same leadership structure. The surgery sections are as follows:

Surgery Section I: Orthognathic surgery, Infection, TMJ, Pathology

Surgery Section II: Trauma, Implants, Reconstruction, Dentoalveolar surgery

Surgery Section III: Adult medical assessment and anesthesia, Pediatric medical assessment and anesthesia, Anesthetic emergency management, Focused additional short topics

The 3 Surgery sections and the Certification Maintenance Section are led by a senior and a junior co-chair. Each year a junior co-chair is appointed to the section for a 2-year term. The co-chairs are assisted by a section editor within each of the sections, who is responsible for reviewing and editing all written examination content. Section editors are appointed to a 2-year term. Expert consultation across the broad scope of oral and maxillofacial surgery is provided to the section editors and co-chairs by content experts in each section.

ITEM WRITING COMMITTEE

New board examiners are selected after a self-nomination process each year and spend at least 2 years assigned to the Item Writing Committee. Selection to the committee is made after

Box 2
Oral certifying examination

I. Medical assessment and management of the surgical patient
   A. Cardiovascular
   B. Pulmonary
   C. Musculoskeletal and nervous system
   D. Endocrine, GI, GU, metabolic
   E. Behavioral and psychiatric
   F. Allergy, immunology, and hematology

II. Anesthesia and analgesia
   A. Local anesthesia
   B. Deep sedation/general anesthesia
   C. Multimodal analgesia
   D. Adult and pediatric office-based anesthetic emergencies

III. Dentoalveolar
   A. Erupted/unerupted teeth
   B. Dentoalveolar injuries
   C. Infections
   D. Soft tissue procedures

IV. Trauma
   A. Evaluation of the patient with trauma
   B. Mandibular injuries
   C. Mid/upper facial injuries
   D. Soft tissue injuries

V. Orthognathic/cleft/OSA
   A. Mandibular deformities
   B. Maxillary deformities
   C. Cleft lip and palate
   D. Craniofacial anomalies
   E. Obstructive sleep apnea

VI. Cosmetic
   A. Nasal
   B. Periorbital, upper/midface
   C. Facial contour alteration
   D. Soft tissue procedures

VII. Temporomandibular disorders/facial pain
   A. Muscular disorders, facial pain
   B. Internal derangements
   C. Degenerative joint disease
   D. Joint reconstruction

VIII. Pathology
   A. Benign lesions of hard tissue
   B. Benign lesions of soft tissue
   C. Infectious, inflammatory, and autoimmune conditions
   D. Salivary gland pathology
   E. Malignant lesions of hard tissue
   F. Malignant lesions of soft tissue

IX. Reconstruction
   A. Nonvascularized hard tissue grafts
   B. Nonvascularized soft tissue grafts
   C. Vascularized grafts
   D. Pedicle flap

X. Implants
   A. Biology and treatment planning
   B. Prosthetic considerations
   C. Hard and soft tissue adjunctive measures
   D. Surgical technique
   E. Complications

XI. Technologies and materials
   A. Imaging
   B. Surgical technologies
   C. Tissue engineering

considering letters of recommendation, letter of interest, scope of practice, and region of the country (for equity on the Examination Committee). Regional advisors to the board are responsible for collecting self-nominations, reviewing/interviewing the applications, and submitting a recommendation to the BOD. The BOD then appoints candidates to the Item Writing Committee for a period of 2 years; numbers of candidates appointed may vary according to the needs of the committee.

ORAL CERTIFYING EXAMINATION COMMITTEE

The Oral Certifying Examination Committee consists of approximately 75 examiners (selected from successful individuals from the Item Writing Committee). Committee responsibilities include case development for and administration of the oral examinations. Examination Committee members are placed in "sections" based on areas of expertise and needs of the committee. Committee members in good standing typically serve a 6-year term but may be invited back with 1-year renewals based on needs of the Board.

Box 3
Certificates of added qualifications: pediatric craniomaxillofacial surgery (Cleft and Craniofacial)

Cleft surgery

  General considerations

  - Patient evaluation
  - Feeding considerations
  - Presurgical orthodontic/orthopedic treatment
  - Interdisciplinary management

  Cleft lip repair

  - Unilateral cleft lip repair
  - Bilateral cleft lip repair
  - Primary nasal reconstruction
  - Complications

  Cleft palate repair

  - Palate repair techniques
  - Intravelar veloplasty
  - Fistula management and repair
  - Complications

  Management of velopharyngeal insufficiency

  - Preoperative assessment
  - Surgical techniques

  Bone graft reconstruction of the cleft maxilla

  - Presurgical orthodontic and orthopedic treatment
  - Surgical techniques
  - Unilateral cleft bone graft
  - Bilateral cleft bone graft
  - Bone harvesting techniques

  Orthognathic surgery in the patient with cleft lip and palate

  - Diagnosis and treatment planning
  - Surgical techniques
  - Complications

  Secondary reconstructive procedures

  - Lip revision
  - Nasal revision and rhinoplasty
  - Adjunctive surgical procedures

Craniofacial surgery

  General considerations:

  - Patient evaluation
  - Diagnostic imaging
  - Treatment planning

  Nonsynostotic (deformational) plagiocephaly

  - Diagnosis
  - Nonsurgical treatment of plagiocephaly
  - Torticollis evaluation and management

  Nonsyndromic craniosynostosis

  - Diagnosis
  - Surgical techniques
  - Complications

  Craniofacial dysostosis syndromes

  - Genetics
  - Diagnosis
  - Surgical techniques and management
  - Stages of reconstruction
  - Complications

  Secondary reconstructive procedures

  - Surgery for secondary dysmorphology
  - Intracranial pressure management
  - Repair of cranial vault defects
  - Complications

  Associated conditions

    Hemifacial microsomia
    Treacher Collins syndrome
    Pierre-Robin sequence
    Other syndromes
    Genetic considerations

TEST DEVELOPMENT

Examination items are written by Item Writing Committee members, surgeons with a scope of practice commiserate with ABOMS standards, and diplomates in good standing with the board. Items are submitted through and maintained within a secure database. Item writers follow specific guidelines in question creation to help ensure a psychometrically valid examination. Among these guidelines are the following:

1. Each item has a stem, a single correct answer, and 3 distractors (incorrect answers).
2. Punctuation must be correct.
3. Items are supported by 2 published references that should be contemporary (within the last 5 years).
4. The difficulty level and practice orientation should be appropriate to the examination being given.

Box 4
Certificates of added qualifications: head and neck oncologic and reconstructive surgery

Pathology

A. Benign lesions of hard tissue

    (Odontogenic tumors, vascular lesions)

B. Salivary gland

    (Minor and major salivary gland tumors)

C. Malignant lesions of hard tissue

    (Sarcomas of the facial skeleton, squamous cell carcinoma of the jaws, metastatic lesions)

D. Malignant lesions of soft tissue

    (Melanoma and nonmelanoma skin cancer, oral and oropharyngeal squamous cell carcinoma, thyroid and parathyroid tumors, vascular lesions, neural lesions, metastatic lesions)

E. Chemoradiation

    (Induction chemotherapy, concomitant chemoradiation therapy, Intensity-Modulated Radiation Therapy, the unknown primary cancer, nasopharyngeal and hypopharyngeal cancer)

Reconstruction

A. Nonvascularized grafts

B. Free vascularized flaps

C. Pedicle flaps

After items have been submitted, each is reviewed by experts in the field whom the BOD has assigned the title *Content Expert*. The questions are checked for relevance, accuracy, and adherence to the blueprint. Once approved by the content expert, the items are forwarded to the board consultant (member of the BOD responsible for the surgery section) and reviewed one more time.

When the time comes to select items for the various written examinations, the IT vendor contracted with the Board will select items according to the blueprint.

PSYCHOMETRICS

Following each examination administration, items are reviewed by a psychometrician to help ensure validity and relevance. Analyses include standard setting and criterion validity, attenuation studies, differential item functioning analysis, forensic data analysis, pass rate trends, test time analysis, validation studies, and drift analysis. Because the examinations are all criterion-referenced assessments, it is possible for every examination taker to pass the examinations. ABOMS examinations are neither graded on curves nor do they automatically fail a percentage of test takers. Examinees are given the opportunity to comment on items after the examination, and these comments are all reviewed by the Directors of the Board.

CERTIFICATION MAINTENANCE

Certification maintenance is the career-long phase of Diplomate Status that annually renews one's commitment to the highest standards of patient care. This commitment is supported by the diplomates continuing education, adherence to the Canons, credential maintenance in one's local community, and the demonstration of clinical acumen and practice improvement standards.

Beginning in 2020, all diplomates with time-limited certificates began the new Certification Maintenance Program. The program is a 10-year cycle that incorporates 4 domains.

1. Evidence of professional standing
2. Evidence of lifelong learning and self-assessment
3. Evidence of cognitive expertise
4. Evaluation of performance in practice

Each year, diplomates verify professional standing by attesting to licensure, continuing education requirements, and hospital privileges. Diplomates are required to review 2 publications selected by the Board and answer review questions on the articles. Every 3 years, diplomates are also required to review 2 clinical case scenarios and answer examination-type questions about the described patient management. Every 5 years, diplomates must report to the BOD on quality improvement initiatives that they have undertaken in their clinical practice (**Fig. 1**).

THOUGHTS ON THE FUTURE

The ABOMS strives to continue to remain contemporary in content of examinations, philosophy of testing, and certification maintenance. By providing updated and referenced examination items and practices that ensure diversity of thought on the committee as well as committee member turnover, the ABOMS will continue to ensure that the public can continue to place trust in the fact that diplomates of the ABOMS provide the most empathetic, professional, and up-to-date care available in the provision of oral and maxillofacial surgery. By providing Certificates of

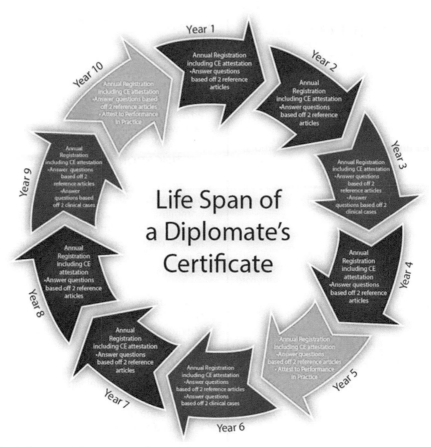

Fig. 1. ■ Life Cycle of a Diplomate's Certificate

Added Qualifications, the ABOMS ensures that the specialty will be able to continue to support the Diplomates who continue their training and expand their scope in the pursuit of excellence.

DISCLOSURE

The authors have nothing to disclose. V.J. Perciaccante: President of the American Board of Oral and Maxillofacial Surgery. L.L. Cunningham, Jr.: Immediate Past President of the American Board of Oral and Maxillofacial Surgery.

ACKNOWLEDGMENTS

The authors would like to thank Courtney Quinn for her assistance in preparation of this article.

REFERENCES

1. Available at: https://www.aboms.org/application/files/6714/9080/4731/Appendix_XVI-Canons_of_Ethical_Conduct.pdf Accessed 2014.

2. Available at: https://www.aboms.org/application/files/8914/9574/6051/ABOMS_history-addendum_2nd_version_082514.pdf Accessed 2010.

Understanding Health Policy and Its Importance in Residency Education for Oral and Maxillofacial Surgery

Jack A. Harris, DMD[a], Yisi D. Ji, MD, DMD[b],*

KEYWORDS

- Health policy • Oral and maxillofacial surgery • Insurance • Value-based care • Education

KEY POINTS

- Health policy plays a large role in shaping the scope and practice of oral and maxillofacial surgery (OMS); an understanding of health policy and physician reimbursement mechanisms will be useful for surgeons
- The development and implementation of a standardized health policy curriculum in dental school and OMS residency training will better prepare surgeons to understand reimbursement and billing practices
- Avenues of advocacy among OMSs and trainees include Congressional lobbying efforts, the development of national outcomes-driven databases for OMS, and the experimentation of alternative payment models with private insurers

INTRODUCTION

Health policy is playing an increasingly important role in shaping the delivery of surgical care and the reimbursement of surgeons. This article aims to provide a brief purview of the current state of health policy through the lens of oral and maxillofacial surgery (OMS). Methods of integrating health policy education into the training of an OMS and possible avenues for advocacy work will also be discussed. This brief article does not aim to serve as a comprehensive overview of the vast field of health policy; rather, the authors hope to highlight pertinent points to OMS that demand active consideration by the OMS community.

The field of OMS is unique as it borders both medical and dental insurance—a fact that requires consideration when addressing the topic of health policy. As the United States (US) health care system begins to transition away from traditional fee-for-service (FFS) reimbursement models, there are increasing legislative and commercial pressures on physicians and surgeons alike to lower health care costs while also demonstrating the value of their services or procedures.

A BRIEF HISTORY OF INSURANCE AND ORAL AND MAXILLOFACIAL SURGERY

The divide between dentistry and medicine spans multiple decades and can be traced back to the 1930s. This initial splintering of dentistry from the rest of medicine has contributed, in part, to the fragmented scope of practice of OMS and the dichotomous pull and existing tension of private practice OMS and academic OMS.

The origins of medical insurance can be linked back to the 1930s, with the introduction of Blue Cross Blue Shield health plans.[1] In contrast, dental insurance was introduced a decade later in the 1940s with the rise of labor unions.[1] These initial insurance plans were limited in their scope of

Funding: There was no funding for this project.
a Harvard School of Dental Medicine, Boston, MA, USA; b Harvard Medical School, Boston, MA, USA
* Corresponding author. 260 Longwood Avenue, Boston, MA 02215.
E-mail address: ydaisyji1@gmail.com

Oral Maxillofacial Surg Clin N Am 34 (2022) 529–536
https://doi.org/10.1016/j.coms.2022.03.004

coverage, as preapproval was required and caps were placed on the amount of money an insurance plan would pay in total benefits.[1] The greatest divergence in the structure of insurance between medicine and dentistry was in 1965 with the passage of Medicare. At the time, both the American Medical Association (AMA) and the American Dental Association (ADA) lobbied against the inclusion of medicine and dentistry in Medicare, respectively; however, only the ADA succeeded in having dentistry excluded.[2] Since this divergence, dentistry, and aspects of OMS, have continued to be excluded from Medicare and other government-funded plans. As many commercial and third-party insurers decide their coverage based on Medicare, the effects from 1965 are still felt today in third-party plans. Consequently, many OMS procedures, historically deemed to be a part of dentistry, are not covered by major health insurers.

Since 1965, the structure of health insurance has undergone incremental, yet substantial, changes, culminating in the passage of the Affordable Care Act (ACA) in 2010. The ACA marked the inception of a new "value-based care" era, a shift from existing FFS reimbursement mechanisms. Specifically, the ACA introduced measures that would aid in the transition of the US health system into a value-based reimbursement system, which emphasizes financial incentives for physicians to enhance the quality of care. Likewise, the Medicare Access and Children's Health Insurance Program (CHIP) reauthorization act (MACRA) of 2015 continued to develop the value-based reimbursement model by introducing a merit-based incentive system (MIPS) and alternative payment models (APMs).

MEDICARE COVERAGE FOR ORAL AND MAXILLOFACIAL SURGERY PROCEDURES

There are select OMS procedures that are covered by Medicare and third-party medical insurers, such as trauma, head and neck cancer surgery, and infections. Orthognathic surgery has variable coverage that is insurer-dependent. This stems from the aforementioned reasons in the sections above.

Roughly 800 to 900 OMSs opt in to Medicare and accept it as insurance—a fraction of the more than 4000 American Association of Oral and Maxillofacial Surgery (AAOMS) members.[3] As such, OMS procedures account for a very small fraction of claims sent to Medicare each year. OMSs typically do not accept Medicare due to lower reimbursement rates compared with third-party payers or cash-only practices. Furthermore,

academic surgeons, more likely to see complex patients than private practice surgeons, are reimbursed less by Medicare.[4] Medicare regularly updates the valuations of its procedures with surveys sent by professional surgical societies to member surgeons. However, for Medicare to consider re-evaluating the appropriate reimbursement for a specific current procedural terminology (CPT) code, that particular code must meet a certain volume threshold of billed Medicare claims annually.[3] Here, OMSs have found themselves in a conundrum, whereby low reimbursement rates disincentivize surgeons from opting into Medicare. Yet, the only way to increase reimbursement rates in Medicare is to produce enough volume to meet the set threshold of Medicare claims to trigger a re-evaluation of the current reimbursement rate for a given procedure.

RELATIVE VALUE UNITS IN ORAL AND MAXILLOFACIAL SURGERY

For years, physician payment and compensation in OMS have followed a FFS mechanism. This reimbursement scheme, more formally known as the Resource-Based Relative Value Scale (RBRVS), was introduced by the Centers for Medicare and Medicaid Services (CMS) in 1992 to better evaluate the time, effort, and skill required by a practitioner to accomplish a healthcare-related task.[5] At the time, the RBRVS system marked a drastic departure from traditional physician payment models, which compensated physicians based on their "usual, customary, and reasonable" fees.[6]

The RBRVS system created a standardized metric to help determine physician reimbursement, known as the relative value unit (RVU), which allows for the comparison of various procedures across disparate specialties. To assist CMS in assigning and updating RVUs, the AMA founded the Relative Value Scale Update Committee (RUC). Currently, RVUs are calculated from surveys of surgeons conducted by various specialty societies, such as the AAOMS. Each specialty society collates the results of its surveys and makes recommendations to the RUC regarding RVU valuations of individual procedures. The RUC then submits these proposals to CMS to determine physician reimbursement rates nationally. As commercial and private insurance payments are based on the CMS Physician Fee Schedule, the RUC's recommendations have the potential to affect nearly 70% of all physician payments in the US (**Fig. 1**).[5,7]

Currently, the total RVU is determined by 3 main components: (1) physician work RVU (wRVU),

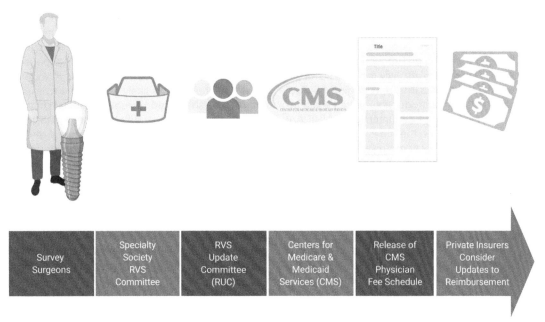

Fig. 1. Figure 1 illustrates the process of developing RVUs for procedures.

which measures the time and skills necessary to perform a given task; (2) practice expense RVU, which measures labor and equipment costs; and (3) professional liability insurance expense RVU, which includes malpractice insurance premiums. Each component of the RVU is geographically adjusted and summed to arrive at the total RVU that can be converted into a dollar amount as determined annually by CMS.

Recent criticisms regarding the RVU system have emerged, particularly regarding the way in which RVUs are calculated. Time estimates, which account for roughly 80% of the variance in wRVUs for a given procedure, are derived from surveys of surgeons with response rates as low as 2.2%.[8] Data from the AMA RBRVS Data Manager have shown similar trends in OMS, with survey response rates of 2.7%.[9] As a result of low response rates, coupled with response bias and individual variability among respondents, these surveys likely fail to accurately represent the true amount of time it takes to complete a procedure. Furthermore, the current rules dictating when RVUs for a given CPT code are to be reviewed and updated by the RUC make it so most of the codes used by OMSs have likely not been reviewed since the 1990s.[9] Recent evaluations of procedural intraoperative times for common OMS procedures, such as head and neck cancer surgeries and infections, have also illustrated discrepancies between CMS estimates and true operating times.[10,11] The accuracy of these surveys in determining RVU valuation is paramount

to OMSs as these values help drive practice patterns in the field and will determine reimbursement rates for surgeons across the US. There have been various proposals to increase the accuracy of CMS' procedural time estimates used in RVU valuation, such as findings ways to increase survey response rates, using clinical repositories such as the American College of Surgeons (ACS) National Surgical Quality Improvement Program (NSQIP) to determine the actual intraoperative time, or developing alternative physician reimbursement models.

RVUs for dental procedures are determined through a similar, albeit slightly different, methodology. Each year, Relative Value Studies Inc. publishes a document titled "Relative Value for Dentists" detailing the base unit RVU valuation of each current dental terminology (CDT) code, which is based on national surveys of dentists and oral health care providers. This base unit RVU valuation is then multiplied by a set monetary conversion factor to arrive at the final compensation for a single CDT code.

MEDICAL AND DENTAL INSURANCE BILLING

A consideration for OMS in terms of properly billing procedures stems from differences in medical and dental coding, which manifests through the use of CPT codes and CDT codes, respectively.[12] The history of the CPT code can be followed back to 1966 with the first publication of the CPT edition of standardized codes by the

AMA with the goal of providing uniformity in billing practices for medical records and insurance.[13] By 1983, CPT codes were adopted as part of the CMS Healthcare Common Procedure Coding System (HCPCS) and were officially recognized as the national standard for billing and coding medical procedures after the introduction of the Health Insurance Portability and Accountability Act (HIPAA) in 1996. CDT codes, on the other hand, were first introduced to the dental community in a 1969 publication in *The Journal of the American Dental Association (JADA)*. Since 1990, the ADA has continually updated CDT codes through the publication of the CDT reference manual, with the CDT code becoming officially recognized as a HIPAA standard code set in 2000.[14]

As OMS lies at the intersection of both medicine and dentistry, OMSs are able to bill services using either the CDT or CPT coding system for select procedures. Whether an OMS bills a procedure as a CPT code or a CDT code typically depends on the nature of the practice and the type of insurance to which the claim will be billed.[15]

PRIVATE PRACTICE ORAL AND MAXILLOFACIAL SURGERY AND HEALTH POLICY

The landscape of private practice OMS has changed over the last several decades and will continue to evolve, accelerated by increasing the acquisition/consolidation of OMS practices by venture capital and private equity firms, the rise of the dental service organization (DSO) and corporate-owned practices, and the introduction of novel reimbursement models.

The attractive financial upside of OMS practices has made them prime targets for buy-outs and acquisitions by DSOs, corporations, and private equity firms, an increasingly common practice as of late.[16–18] Private equity firms have been eager to acquire OMS practices for 3 primary reasons: (1) the market is geographically fragmented, allowing efficient consolidation and management of different practices into a single regional brand, (2) the upside of economies of scale from roll-ups, and (3) the increasing demand for OMS services due to the aging US population.[19] There are several implications that a private practice OMS should evaluate when considering a private equity buy-out. For example, private equity firms can provide large capital investment for equipment and technology as well as manage business operations to reduce the administrative burden of owning a practice. Furthermore, the sale of the practice to the private equity firm is taxed at a capital gains tax, which is typically lower than income tax. However, the acquisition of OMS practices by private equity comes at a cost, namely the loss of surgeon autonomy and the subsequent emphasis on procedural volume at the potential expense of the quality of patient care and safety.[19] Nonetheless, private equity is likely to continue to expand its market share and disrupt traditional methods of OMS care delivery. Whether the expansion of private equity into the private sector will result in an increased value of care is yet to be determined.

VARIOUS REIMBURSEMENT MODELS FOR ORAL AND MAXILLOFACIAL SURGERY

OMSs have traditionally been reimbursed through a FFS mechanism. Despite its lucrative nature, many critics of the FFS model stress that it emphasizes and prioritizes the provision of a greater number of services at the expense of quality.[20] In response, there has been a recent trend toward alternative payment models that incentivize value over volume. Some examples of value-based payment models include bundled payment systems (a physician receives a fixed amount of money for all services related to an episode of care), capitation plans (a provider receives a fixed amount of money for each patient), shared savings models (similar to the FFS model, but the payment is based on quality and spending targets), and shared risk models (spending is encouraged to remain below target rates, with the provider covering all excess costs). Similar to bundled payments for hip and knee replacements in orthopedic surgery, some have proposed that bundled payment models could be adapted for certain procedures in OMS such as total joint replacement of the temporomandibular joint (TMJ).[20,21] The potential benefits of implementing a bundled payment system include a reduction in wasteful spending, shorter hospitalizations, and a reduction in unnecessary hospital admissions. Although there is still much research needed to assess the financial and health-related effects of alternative reimbursement models in OMS, value-based care is likely to impact the future practice of both private and hospital-based surgeons in the coming years.

THE FUTURE OF ORAL AND MAXILLOFACIAL SURGERY

The growing presence of corporate entities as discussed previously leaves innumerable implications for OMSs and patients.[22] As one example and a harbinger of potential future issues, the Attorney General of New York filed a lawsuit against Aspen Dental in 2015 for violating the ban on corporate medicine.[22] In essence, Aspen Dental was placing its corporate interests ahead of its duty to patient care.[22] The suit was ultimately settled with concessions by Aspen Dental to insulate its clinical components from its business component and a civil penalty of $450,000.[22] This is just one example of the commercialization and deprofessionalization of dentistry—driven by venture capital and private equity firms who increasingly possess a larger portion of ownership.[22] OMSs employed by such corporations or acquired by private equity might be placed under similar pressure from management to increase production to meet the dividend returns expected by certain stakeholders. While OMS has traditionally been viewed as a specialty of both medicine and dentistry, the degradation of the divide between private practice dentistry and patient care is in direct conflict with the ethos of medicine and health care.

The decision of whether OMS follows the rest of the dental field in the commercialization of oral health will in part impact the overall trajectory and scope of the field. OMS will have to choose whether it considers itself a commodity on a free market, subject to market forces and acquisitions (as embodied by much of dentistry already), or an essential health service.[23] Criticisms have emerged regarding the field's reliance on the continued popularity of the private practice model and divergence from hospital-based practice.[24] If oral and maxillofacial surgeons continue to favor the private practice model at the expense of hospital affiliation, the profession is likely to relinquish much of the surgical scope that it had previously worked so hard to secure. Undoubtedly, whichever consensus is reached by the field will dictate the future and viability of OMS.

INTEGRATING HEALTH POLICY INTO ORAL AND MAXILLOFACIAL SURGICAL TRAINING

Formal instruction in health systems, insurance, and reimbursement mechanisms has traditionally been excluded as part of the education of a US-trained OMS. At present, the Commission on Dental Accreditation (CODA) for predoctoral dental education does not specifically require dental school curricula to include instruction in oral health policy or health policy at large, despite many dental schools providing courses in practice management and business strategy.[25] While such courses are useful, they are generally taught from the perspective of small-business ownership rather than from a systems approach. Nonetheless, various organizations such as the Public Policy and Advocacy group of the American Dental Education Association (ADEA) and American

Student Dental Association (ASDA) have acknowledged the importance of encouraging dental students to participate in political, legislative, and health policy advocacy work.[26,27] Similarly, CODA does not include health policy education in its accreditation standards for US advanced dental education programs in OMS.[28] Much of the health policy educational materials for OMSs have come in the form of scattered journal articles and short perspective pieces, such as those published by AAOMS.[29]

The development of a standard health policy curriculum in dental school and OMS residency training is long overdue. Dental students would benefit from a foundational purview of health policy principles including health systems, finance and insurance structures, quality improvement and patient safety, health disparities, health care advocacy, politics, and law, continuing with further training, didactics, and application during OMS residency training. As trainees advance in their education, the relevant knowledge of health policy and insurance would ideally complement their clinical experiences. For example, residents frequently interact with Medicare and Medicaid patients during their residency training. Providing didactic supplementation on how their procedures (eg, mandible fractures, incision, and drainage of abscesses, etc.) are reimbursed allows trainees to gain perspective on how these procedures may or may not complement their future scope of practice. Specifically, attending surgeons could require trainees at the end of each operation to determine how they would bill each procedure and if they would use any modifiers (ie, for complexity/time). Such active integration of health policy and billing principles into surgical training will better prepare trainees when they enter independent practice.

The implementation of a standardized health policy curriculum is crucial due to the heterogeneity in dental school education and OMS residency training throughout the US. The authors propose a framework for a health policy curriculum to be integrated into the educational training of an OMS (**Table 1**). While some of these topics may seem abstract to the budding dental student, core principles can be revisited during residency training at various iterations and in greater depth as trainees become more nuanced and subspecialized. Furthermore, surgical residents are best equipped to reinforce and apply didactic principles having interacted with the health care system first-hand. Subsequently, health policy will no longer become an abstract theoretical framework, but instead an overarching theme with practical implications that seeps into their day-to-day practice.[30]

Table 1
A proposed health policy curricular framework for OMS education

Educational Pillars	Core Concepts
1. Population and Public Health	Social Determinants of Health Health Disparities Disease Prevention Health Improvement Health care Advocacy
2. Health Care Delivery and Economics	Health care Delivery Processes and Structures Collaboration and Coordination of Health care Delivery Economic Policy Physician Reimbursement Insurance Models
3. Value-Based Care	Quality Principles and Metrics Quality Improvement Evaluation and Metrics Efficiency and Waste Institute of Medicine's Dimensions of Quality Gaps in Health care Delivery
4. Systems Approach	Multi-Directional Cause-Effect Relationships Complex System Interdependencies
5. Ethics, Politics, and Law	Codes of Conduct Ethics and Professionalism Government Policy and Law

Data from Gonzalo JD, Dekhtyar M, Starr SR, Borkan J, Brunett P, Fancher T, Green J, Grethlein SJ, Lai C, Lawson L, Monrad S, O'Sullivan P, Schwartz MD, Skochelak S. Health Systems Science Curricula in Undergraduate Medical Education: Identifying and Defining a Potential Curricular Framework. Acad Med. 2017 Jan;92(1):123-131.

As technologies and health care infrastructures evolve, so too must the delivery of information and educational platforms to trainees. With the abundant didactic and clinical obligations of dental students and OMS resident trainees and subsequent time constraints, it is essential that nontraditional educational platforms be created to facilitate learning outside of structured curricular time. With OMS residency programs already struggling to meet the 30 months of CODA-required OMS clinical training, it is unlikely that a formal health policy curriculum could be incorporated into residency training. Instead, the authors suggest the development of an open-access resource for health policy education in OMS. A similar concept already exists in medicine, known as "Free Open-Access Medical education" (FOAMed), which includes blogs, podcasts, tweets, online videos, text documents, Facebook groups, photographs, and many other forms of interactive open-access medical educational resources designed to supplement traditional educational platforms. Emergency medicine has conducted particularly well with incorporating FOAMed into their curriculum.[31] Many of their websites are now common resources for both emergency medicine residents and also residents of other specialties who might interface with similar topics, such as electrocardiogram (ECG) interpretation. A similar resource could be developed for OMS trainees, which could include open-access videos, written explanations, and health policy podcasts specifically tailored toward dental students and OMS residents to allow for flexibility and adaptation to the trainee's schedule. These resources could further serve to provide continuing education (CE) credit for practicing surgeons.

Admittedly, numerous barriers exist to implementing health policy education throughout oral and maxillofacial surgical training. For example, many trainees will consider this topic to be extraneous as they are focused primarily on the acquisition of technical skills. The authors argue that while technical skills will prepare trainees to be excellent technicians, a robust education in health policy principles will better allow OMSs to thrive and adapt to changing health care landscapes, and ultimately be more successful in their practice. An understanding of billing and reimbursement systems will better equip OMSs to accurately and efficiently bill for services rendered. Further, the introduction of additional didactic requirements into an already overwhelmed and time-restricted residency program may place an undue burden on trainees. As such, the implementation of a health policy curriculum must take into account the time restraints of trainees. Educators can develop novel educational tools, such as FOAMed, which will allow trainees to learn at their pace. Lastly, there has been scarce literature regarding the design and implementation of a health policy curriculum dedicated to OMS. As such, future research efforts should focus on establishing a validated pedagogy aimed at developing a foundation in health policy during dental school education and continuing throughout residency training. Possible avenues of addressing this limitation are to learn from what our medical colleagues have conducted in terms of developing and implementing a health policy into the medical school curriculum.

AVENUES FOR ADVOCACY BY TRAINEES

Traditional methods of advocacy include lobbying legislative cohorts at the state or federal level through various professional and nonprofessional organizations. For example, AAOMS frequently participates in lobbying Congress on legislative bills that affect OMSs. This may be the most common avenue for interested surgeons and surgical trainees to become involved in advocacy work.

Other lesser known methods of affecting change include partnering with private insurers to pilot new payment models or methods of delivering care. As an example, in February 2020 Blue Cross Blue Shield partnered with a private practice dental group and announced the nation's first value-based payment model for dentistry.[32,33] Under this new model, dental providers who demonstrate improvements in their patient's oral and systemic health, based on set metrics, will receive an incentive payment. For example, patients with diabetes and coronary artery disease would receive more frequent prophylactic oral health care such as dental cleanings and periodontal treatments aimed at improving the systemic health outcomes in these particular individuals. A similar partnership could be developed between OMS practices and private insurers, allowing for the delivery of alternative payment models such as bundled payment systems, shared savings/risk plans, and global capitation. This method of health policy advocacy allows surgeons to have direct input on how they are reimbursed and may be less circuitous than traditional lobbying efforts.

Finally, the development of a national outcomes-driven database for OMS procedures will be critical in health policy advocacy and ensuring fair compensation for OMS procedures. Assertions on fair reimbursement for surgical procedures are increasingly met with requests for objective evidence justifying such costs. The field of general surgery has developed multiple national databases, such as the National Trauma Database (NTDB) and NSQIP datasets, which permit surgeons to demonstrate improved patient outcomes, safety, and lower costs—highlighting the value of surgical care. While some studies in OMS have been published piggybacking on the existing NSQIP datasets, much of the NSQIP data are not specific to OMS and is lacking in granularity of OMS-specific outcomes. In addition, the outcomes of many NSQIP-related "OMS" procedures are typically performed by either general surgeons, plastic surgeons, or otolaryngologists. By having OMS-specific data, surgeons would be able to provide evidence-based literature justifying the value of surgical care provided. Nonetheless, very few studies of this nature exist in OMS, and the few studies available demonstrating the value of OMS procedures are of admittedly poor quality.[34]

SUMMARY

A fundamental understanding of health policy is necessary for OMSs to take part in actively shaping the ever-changing landscape of health insurance and to help ensure fair reimbursement for OMS procedures. The incorporation of standardized health policy curricula in the training of an OMS will be essential in helping surgeons shape their future practice.

DISCLOSURE

The authors have no conflicts of interest to disclose.

ACKNOWLEDGMENTS

The authors would like to thank Dr. Eric R. Carlson DMD MD FACS for his guidance and insight.

REFERENCES

1. Simon L. Overcoming Historical Separation between Oral and General Health Care: Interprofessional Collaboration for Promoting Health Equity. AMA J Ethics 2016;18:941.
2. Ji YD, Peacock ZS, Dodson TB. Political Preferences of Oral and Maxillofacial Surgeons: The Elephant (and Donkey) in the Room. J Oral Maxillofac Surg 2019;77:1105.
3. Ji YD, Peacock ZS, Hupp JR. Medicare in Oral and Maxillofacial Surgery: Disparities in Access Part 1. J Oral Maxillofac Surg 2018;76:1837.
4. Ji YD, Peacock ZS, Hupp JR. Medicare in Oral and Maxillofacial Surgery Part 2: Academic Surgeons

and Cancer Surgeons Are Reimbursed Less. J Oral Maxillofac Surg 2019;77:698.

5. Urwin JW, Gudbranson E, Graham D, et al. Accuracy Of The Relative Value Scale Update Committee's Time Estimates And Physician Fee Schedule For Joint Replacement. Health Aff 2019;38:1079.

6. Glaser WA. The politics of paying American physicians. Health Aff 1989;8:129.

7. Urwin JW, Emanuel EJ. The Relative Value Scale Update Committee: Time for an Update. JAMA 2019;322(12):1137–8.

8. Chan DC, Huynh J, Studdert DM. Accuracy of Valuations of Surgical Procedures in the Medicare Fee Schedule. N Engl J Med 2019;380:1546.

9. Harris JA, Ji YD, McCain JP. Accuracy of the Relative Value Units in Oral and Maxillofacial Surgery. J Oral Maxillofac Surg 2021;79:7.

10. Harris JA, McCain JP, Carlson ER, et al. Assessment of Intraoperative Time for Head and Neck Cancer Surgeries Compared With Medicare Work Time. J Oral Maxillofac Surg 2021;79:483.

11. Harris JA, McCain JP, Untrauer JB, et al. Evaluation of Procedural Intraoperative Time for Head and Neck Infections: Impact on Surgeon Reimbursement. J Oral Maxillofac Surg 2021;79:14.

12. Code on Dental Procedures and Nomenclature (CDT Code). American Dental Association. Available at: https://www.ada.org/en/publications/cdt. Accessed October 30, 2021.

13. Dotson P. CPT® Codes: What Are They, Why Are They Necessary, and How Are They Developed? Adv Wound Care 2013;2:583.

14. Standard Terminologies and Codes. American Dental Association. Available at: https://www.ada.org/en/member-center/member-benefits/practice-resources/dental-informatics/standard-terminologies-and-codes. Accessed October 30, 2021.

15. Rohde S. The Who, What, When and How of Dental Codes. EideBailly. Available at: https://www.eidebailly.com/insights/articles/2019/9/dental-coding. Accessed October 30, 2021.

16. Affinity Has Now Added Oral Surgery to its Expansive Multi-Specialty Platform. MidOcean Partners. Available at: https://www.midoceanpartners.com/news-media/2019-09-20-affinity-has-now-added-oral-surgery-to-its-expansive-multi-specialty-platform. Accessed October 25, 2021.

17. RiverGlade Capital Announces the Formation of U.S. Oral Surgery Management. RiverGlade Capital. Available at: https://rivergladecapital.com/us-oral-surgery-management/. Accessed October 25, 2021.

18. Wall Street Transforms Dentistry Into a Credit-Fueled Gold Rush. Bloomberg. Available at: https://www.bloomberg.com/news/articles/2018-06-28/wall-street-transforms-dentistry-into-a-credit-fueled-gold-rush. Accessed October 25, 2021.

19. Patel NA, Afshar S. Implications of Private Equity in Oral and Maxillofacial Surgery. J Oral Maxillofac Surg 2020;78:1456.

20. Patel NA, Ji YD, McCain JP, et al. Alternative Payment Models in Oral and Maxillofacial Surgery: A Proposal for Bundled Payments for Total Joint Replacements. J Oral Maxillofac Surg 2019;77:2175.

21. Comprehensive Care for Joint Replacement Model. Centers for Medicare & Medicaid Services. Available at: https://innovation.cms.gov/innovation-models/cjr. Accessed October 30, 2021.

22. 'eel Cajee N. Disruptures in the Dental Ethos: The Birth, Life, & Neoliberal Retirement of Norms in Advertising & Corporatization. J L Med Ethics 2021;49:77.

23. Simon L. From Exceptionalism to Essentialism in Dentistry. J L Med Ethics 2021;49:89.

24. Hupp JR. Retreating to our cottages. Oral Surg Oral Med Oral Pathol Oral Radiol Endod 2005;99:391.

25. Commission on Dental Accreditation: Accreditation Standards For Dental Education Programs., 2021.

26. Bresch JE, Luke GG, McKinnon MD, et al. Today's threat is tomorrow's crisis: advocating for dental education, dental and biomedical research, and oral health. J Dent Educ 2006;70:601.

27. Bensch B. Dental students–dental advocates. J Am Coll Dent 2010;77(14).

28. Commission on Dental Accreditation: Accreditation Standards for Advanced Dental Education Programs in Oral and Maxillofacial Surgery., 2021.

29. American Association of Oral and Maxillofacial Surgeons: 2015 Medicare Physician Quality Reporting System (PQRS). AAOMS Today 2015;13:4.

30. Gonzalo JD, Dekhtyar M, Starr SR, et al. Health Systems Science Curricula in Undergraduate Medical Education: Identifying and Defining a Potential Curricular Framework. Acad Med 2017;92:123.

31. Library • LITFL Medical Blog • Life in the Fast Lane. Life In The Fast Lane. 2020. Available at: https://litfl.com/library/. Accessed May 25, 2021.

32. Cryts A. Massachusetts Blues Plan Signs Nation's First Value-Based Care Contract with Dental Management Group. Available at: https://www.managedhealthcareexecutive.com/view/massachusetts-blues-plan-signs-nations-first-value-based-care-contract-dental-management. Accessed May 14, 2021.

33. Blue Cross Blue Shield Of Massachusetts Announces Innovative Value-Based Partnership With Dental Management Company 42 North. Available at: https://newsroom.bluecrossma.com/2020-02-25-Blue-Cross-Blue-Shield-Of-Massachusetts-Announces-Innovative-Value-Based-Partnership-With-Dental-Management-Company-42-North. Accessed May 14, 2021.

34. Geisler BP, Ji YD, Peacock ZS. Value in Oral and Maxillofacial Surgery: A Systematic Review of Economic Analyses. J Oral Maxillofac Surg 2017;75:2287.

Residency Education in Oral and Maxillofacial Surgery: A New Curriculum Framework

Leon A. Assael, DMD[a,b,c],*

KEYWORDS

- Education • Oral and maxillofacial surgery • The quadruple aim • Core competencies • Milestones
- Workforce

KEY POINTS

- The Oral Health in America Report of the National Institutes of Health and actions of the American Council on Graduate Medical Education are recrafting a new framework for structuring and adapting oral and maxillofacial surgery (OMS) programs.
- Advances in surgical technology, the public use (and misuse) of formerly arcane and sequestered medical information, and social media's acceleration toward the Metaverse are a few of the trends that will transform OMS surgical education.
- Essential understanding of oral diseases and observations made in primary care medical settings, taught in part in the academic medical setting by OMS, can substantially bridge the medical/dental divide in health.
- Achieving the quadruple aim in OMS practice: improving the patient care experience, improved population health outcomes, cost efficiency in health care, with a good health care team experience is a concept that must be initiated and promulgated in our residency programs.

Although residents, program directors, and faculty may consider oral and maxillofacial surgery (OMS) residencies as stable and unfettered bastions, every program now exists in an environment of transformation unlike anything in the past in the United States. Changes in American society accelerated by the COVID-19 pandemic are impacting health-care education and demanding a comprehensive understanding and response in our programs and standards.

Profound changes in higher education in the United States are now impacting surgical education, dental education, medical education, and the university education. Due to its position in the hospital as a certificate program, OMS residency education has remained somewhat insulated from the brunt of these changes, until now. Changes in the medical school curriculum are requiring a considered and substantial response in the construct of MD integrated programs. OMS curriculum and the structure and function of residency programs will soon transform to accommodate this environment and, perhaps, to benefit from it. The affiliated universities and their dental schools are in a new landscape of financial responsibility and societal relevance. The accreditation standards of the Commission on Dental Accreditation (CODA) are as well being influenced by the US Department of Education and the political landscape to reflect this changing environment.

Advances in surgical technology, the public use (and misuse) of formerly arcane and sequestered medical information, and social media's acceleration toward the Metaverse are a few of the trends that will transform OMS surgical education. Multiple users of medical information: the public, payers, lawyers, business leaders, social media

^a Department of Restorative and Preventive Dentistry, University of California San Francisco; ^b University of Minnesota; ^c Oral and Maxillofacial Surgery, Oregon Health & Science University
* 8150 Northeast Hidden Cove Road, Bainbridge Island, WA 98110.
E-mail addresses: leonassael@gmail.com; leon.assael@ucsf.edu

Oral Maxillofacial Surg Clin N Am 34 (2022) 537–544
https://doi.org/10.1016/j.coms.2022.03.009
1042-3699/22/© 2022 Elsevier Inc. All rights reserved.

influencers, decision makers, surgeons, faculty, staff, and so forth are all accessing the same informatics/social media environment creating currents that effect care and surgical education in, as yet, unimaginable ways.

These changes in the characteristics of the US public, the demands of patient care, the altered epidemiology of OMS diseases, and the perceived public need for care are evolving in ways that do not match the current structure of clinical education in OMS. The purpose of this article is to consider some of those major transformations and how OMS residencies might react to them and thereby improve OMS education.

ORAL HEALTH IN AMERICA: IMPLICATIONS FOR ORAL AND MAXILLOFACIAL SURGERY EDUCATION

The NIDCR has influenced our understanding of trends in oral diseases with the publication of Oral Health in America: Advances and Challenges, a 20-year follow-up on the surgeon's general report on oral health.[1] The report describes how a greater understanding of the oral microbiome has given a detailed analysis of the pathogenesis, prevention, and treatment of the 3 major oral diseases: caries, periodontal disease, and oral cancer. It describes the need for oral health education to integrate its programs and workforce into an interprofessional practice setting, along with a common electronic health record, and integrated medical/dental practice models. The report indicates the inexorable role that oral health must play in advancing health in America.

The implications of this report for OMS education are enormous. This begins with an understanding that OMS residencies stand as the single greatest oral health education resource to further the aims of this report. Currently, OMS departments in academic health centers advance the goals of this report, with its integrated dental/medical education model, its essential role in trauma and oncology care, and educational programs that are comfortable as an integrated component of graduate health sciences education. In addition, OMS residencies have the opportunity to further their role as educational resources to medical surgical residencies and medical schools, most importantly in those medical specialties that have the greatest impact on health: primary care, pediatrics, and behavioral health. Essential understanding of oral diseases and observations made in primary care medical settings, taught in part in the academic medical setting by OMS, can substantially bridge the medical/dental divide in health.[2]

The report indicates that in the United States, gains in oral health have advanced, then stalled. Gains have been due to advances in the understanding of the pathogenesis, and subsequent treatment of major oral diseases. As examples, minimally invasive caries management, remineralization, as well as therapy altering the microbiome are substantially reducing tooth loss with further gains to come. However, further advancement of technology and workforce are *not* the current principal barriers to achieving further gains in oral health.

Oral health disparities now produce most oral disease and untreated/inadequately treated disease among all causes. Oral health is now achieved due mostly to overcoming social and economic factors, not technological or biological factors. Simply, oral health disparities are due mainly to the financial barriers to achieving oral health. These barriers are produced, importantly, not only by individual finances but also by public policy decisions such as the exclusion of dental services in Medicare, cultural barriers, and family structure barriers. To consider the impact of these societal changes, address the issue of elective third molar removal, which depends strongly on a patient with private dental insurance who use those services. Today a greater number of Americans than ever, including a greater number of minorities have private medical and dental insurance.[3] Yet there has been a continuous decline in utilization of oral health care services in adults since the Great Recession.[4] Although the impact of these factors exists in all aspects of health care, it is greatest in oral health. Vujicic and colleagues, at the American Dental Association Center for Health Policy has documented that dental care presents the single greatest financial barrier to patients among all health services.[5]

Although OMS residencies cannot do more than accommodate to this environment of poor access to care, education in OMS must see itself as an essential asset in addressing oral health disparities and the other findings of the Oral Health in America National Institute of Dental and Craniofacial Research (NIDCR) report. Existing tools in clinical education and practice can be used to advance access to care. As a means to influence clinical practice, OMS residencies must respond by providing care that reduces the patient's financial burden in pursuit of improved patient outcomes (the Quadruple Aim). In addition, using the American Council on Graduate Medical Education (ACGME) core competencies for resident education for example, for "systems based practice" can be a means of teaching and practicing improved health outcomes through navigation of a complex system of health care delivery. By demonstrating the value of OMS care to the patient, the demand curve for OMS services will improve positively influencing patients and health-care system decisions. Although not an obvious contention, the OMS curriculum is a key tool in that effort.

A NEW FRAMEWORK FOR ORAL AND MAXILLOFACIAL SURGERY CURRICULUM
The Quadruple Aim

Achieving the quadruple aim in OMS practice: improving the patient care experience, improved population health outcomes, cost efficiency in health care, with a good health care team experience is a concept that must be initiated and promulgated in our residency programs. In the didactic program, case conferences can be used to explore care options and assess outcomes based on the features of the quadruple aim. Departmental care audits that look at length of stay, operating room time, readmissions, complications, and other typical quality measures can examine progress in the quadruple aim as a multifactorial evaluation. Assessing the satisfaction with the care model of both patients and the care team (residents, faculty, and staff), using verifiable survey tools, can be used to improve according to program-specific quadruple aim benchmarks that can be initiated and evolved.[6] Simulation models using standardized cases can support understanding of the care team in making evidence-based decisions that support these goals.

As a simple example, a critical question in OMS residency training might be whether closed reduction and maxillomandibular fixation or open reduction with stable internal fixation is better treatment of a given mandible fracture. A quadruple aim-oriented case conference addressing this would consider which method provides a better patient experience with regard to pain, activities of daily living, patient safety, return to work, and so forth. Which method is better with regard to cost, length of stay, operating room time need for readmission/reoperation, and so forth? Which method can be provided in a variety of settings across populations that might require such treatment? What are the care team knowledge and skill needs for each method? Which method provides the safest and most satisfying team experience? The quadruple aims provide a useful framework to build quality and critically assess clinical care in OMS residencies. It can provide a lifelong framework for residents in clinical decision-making.

The quadruple aim can thus be considered as a framework for components of the didactic program of OMS residencies. Components of the teaching program that are influenced by the quadruple aim include the following:

1. Improving the patient experience: Programs should review their teaching (in the clinical setting and with supporting didactics), of history taking, motivational interviewing, delivering difficult information to the patient, family dynamics in health care, cultural awareness, child life programs, step down services, discharge planning, rehab services, dietary counseling, smoking cessation, and pain control/opioid use. These curriculum components can all be framed around improving the patient experience and thereby producing more effective care outcomes.

2. Cost efficiency: Didactics in the economics of point of service care, ambulatory surgery, operating room efficiency, minimally invasive care, a balanced approach in assessing health outcomes, and evidence-based medical decisions are, in part, framed around the cost of care. Providing an understanding that clinical care decisions produce a cost/benefit to patients and health systems is a necessary analysis for OMS education. Understanding that all diagnostic and treatment plans whether for elective or urgent treatment depend on cost analysis is a difficult but essential lesson for trainees.

3. Population health: The robust team needed to care for oral cancer, craniofacial trauma, mass pandemics, craniofacial disorders, and oral facial pain among others must be taught in the context of community need. Where are such centers needed and how are they structured to respond effectively? How is OMS an essential component of population health in those teams? How do OMS surgical interventions positively influence communities and economies? Understanding population health trends will help direct educational content as in the examples of Human Papilloma Virus (HPV)-related head and neck cancer, use of antiosteoclastic drugs, or the opioid epidemic.

4. The health-care team experience: As an addition to the triple aim, health-care policy makers are finally recognizing that the health-care team is being adversely affected in today's complex health systems. Although the effects of the COVID 19 pandemic are obvious, demands in the logistics of health-care education such as the enormous human energy expenditure of the electronic health record, accreditation of hospitals and residencies, as well as the oversight of regulators have placed exceptional strain on the health-care team in the

years leading up to the pandemic. This has resulted in a steady increase in burnout, career change, and early retirement.[7] Resident faculty and staff wellness, avoiding burnout, alcohol and substance abuse, mental health resources, the exigencies of dealing in uncertainty and failure in clinical practice,[8] building a constructive and effective care team are components of didactics that can complement the other goals of the quadruple aim. Periodic department wide didactic conferences, including clinical, research, laboratory, and clerical staff can support clinical care improvements, whereas building a more effective team. Institution wide programs can further address these issues but only with the active participation of the OMS team.

ACGME Core Competencies

The ACGME core competencies were developed to provide a framework for all graduate medical education programs to achieve their objectives both for the program and for individual residents. They recognize that there are common components to all physician education that must be achieved in creating a capable clinician. ACGME core competencies provide a checklist for the components of residency education that should be incorporated into all components of the educational program. To review, The American Council on Graduate Medical Education promulgated the core competencies for physician training in 1999. These are considered to be essential common components of all residency and fellowship programs and are in current use across more than 135 program types.[9] Unfortunately, these remain to be embraced in graduate dental education or by CODA accreditation of OMS programs.

Although the American Dental Education Association adopted competencies for the new general dentist in 2008 (including the domains of critical thinking, professionalism, communication and interpersonal skills, health promotion, practice management and informatics, and patient care), these are not sufficient to match the needs of our hospital-based, health systems integrated OMS residencies.[10] ACGME core competencies are a current essential need for OMS residency curriculum, program evaluation, and assessing the competencies of enrollees and graduates. Achievement of these competencies can be assessed through the acquisition of Milestones (competency based developmental outcomes: knowledge, skills, attitudes, and performance measures) that can be described throughout training from novice, to unsupervised practice.[11]

The 6 ACGME core-competencies and their relevance to OMS education are as follows:

1. *Practice based learning and improvement*: Dental students have scant experience with practice-based learning in that they are educated mostly in student-based clinics. For the first time in their education, OMS Post Graduate Year (PGY)1 residents become a part of a care team that must provide patient-centered, efficient, and effective care. Graduates of OMS programs must have achieved milestones that position them to lead such practices. To achieve this, the best-positioned OMS residencies are those that create ideal practice models, across the spectrum of societal and clinical need, and led by faculty clinicians with exceptional clinical and leadership capacity.

2. *Patient care and procedural skills*: OMS education remains strongly focused on the development of these skills but is just now coming to terms with how to measure them. A framework of entrusted professional activities (EPAs) is under consideration but is yet to be constructed in OMS. In orthopedics, a list of 285 EPAs were made and consolidated to 49.[12] These must now undergo peer review for validity and subsequently the development of milestones for achieving these EPAs. In pediatric medicine, the Pediatric Milestone Project is identifying and validating EPAs for the purpose of creating a framework useful for resident assessment, resident progression, appointment and privileging, program assessment, and accreditation.[13] Subsequently, development plus validation of the outcomes of the EPA and milestone program must be made for OMS. This is an enormous task for any specialty but it might provide the only reasonable pathway for truly assessing patient care and procedural skill.

3. *Systems based practice*: Understanding health payment systems, the organization of hospitals, practices, and other health-care delivery entities, the utilization of the electronic health record and global health systems are among the competencies needed in the OMS resident. Experiential learning in a health systems environment as well as incorporating as learners into OMS practice that are a part of health systems are means of gaining this core OMS competency. Because of its bridging of dental and medical/surgical health systems, this task is particularly vexing for OMS residencies. OMS residents need to improve their understanding of the health systems in which they reside.

Experiential activities with medical boards, quality improvement activities, operating room/ Emergency Department (ED) committees as well as didactic programs on the health system are needed to gain an understanding of the practitioner's role in health systems. Rotations in private and other community-based OMS practices should gain resident understanding of oral health systems as well.

4. *Medical knowledge*: The entire purpose of acquired clinical didactic knowledge is to support a decision affecting the care of a patient. Utilization of didactic knowledge in OMS has been transformed by Informatics, which relies on how the most valid relevant information is acquired and used in preference to how much information is retained. Creating a balance between what knowledge can be recounted by a resident and what can be acquired and used in a valid way in real time is a necessary challenge to support health-care decisions in clinical OMS practice. Knowledge must be sufficient to ask the right clinical questions but it remains an unreliable means of making clinical decisions. Residents must learn to continuously access contemporary knowledge in clinical practice and make evidence-based clinical care decisions using concurrent knowledge affected by their own clinical experience and the experiences of the care team.

5. *Interpersonal and communication skills*: Dental students do not obtain the extensive skills of medical students in patient interviews, history taking, and counseling. Residencies in OMS benefit from introduction to clinical medicine courses as well as medicine rotations to support communication skills. Communication in clinical OMS practice exists not only to obtain and relate information but also to positively influence behavior in patients, colleagues, and the clinical care team. Motivational interviewing, developed by Miller and Rollnick has had a strong contemporary influence on health science education. It is a means of providing a structured directed patient history/interview style that supports goals that improve health: support patient compliance, self-improvement, and patient satisfaction.[14] Communication should have a defined palette of expected outcomes. Operating suite communication, including subjects such as the "pause," surgical site confirmation, clear reciprocal communication of instructions between the surgeon and care team, and the "handoff" are skills that must be continuously practiced and taught.

6. *Professionalism*: Professionalism in our time is a rapidly evolving area and a markedly sensitive one: considering how society is wrestling in a very active way with race, gender, conflict of interest, dual commitment, meaning of consent, economic and social status, nationality, religion, financial responsibility, corporate relations, clinical research ethics, animal research ethics, corporate responsibility, multiculturalism, aggressive behaviors substance abuse, and morality among a panoply of domains that impact professionalism. Although these are currently buffeting all medical surgical training, OMS may be particularly in need of addressing professionalism in a contemporary manner. This is due to the small size of our programs, challenges in sustaining a diverse OMS environment, and the highly specialized role our programs play in medical surgical education. OMS residencies need to access all the programs and capacities of the institution's professionalism education and support programs through the Graduate Medical Education and Medical Staff offices among others. Joint programs across Graduate Medical Education (GME) residencies are needed to support professionalism in OMS programs.

Evolving Clinical Education

Much of CODA clinical education requirements have remained relatively unchanged for decades. Advances in scope of practice for OMS is often occurring beyond the residency programs toward fellowships, most importantly in oncology, reconstruction, cosmetic surgery, trauma, and pediatric/craniofacial OMS. The volume of experience in core areas of OMS education is facing challenges. Needed additional training and ability in implant dentistry, orthognathic surgery, cosmetic surgery, and anesthesia among others have been mostly achieved via continuing medical education.

The requirements for clinical education are driven by CODA requirements and the perceived needs of the practicing community expressed through the American Association of Oral and Maxillofacial Surgeons (AAOMS) and American Board of Oral and Maxillofacial Surgery (ABOMS). This has resulted in challenges and skewing of clinical experiences in OMS programs. For example, ambulatory anesthesia education may not be well matched to the clinical need in our programs for clinical care. Although our CODA standards insist on a high need for pediatric anesthesia services for oral surgery, the need for children to have a general anesthetic for an ambulatory procedure has diminished sharply, especially for very young children. This is due to the sharply diminished prevalence of early childhood caries as well as the higher restoration of primary teeth.[15] Programs are often left to complete the numerical requirement for pediatric cases by providing anesthesia services for non-OMS surgical procedures.

Clinical care in OMS programs and societal/practice needs are often ill matched. For example, although management of edentulism with surgical interventions remains a core requirement of dental education and OMS training in CODA standards, the prevalence of edentulism in the United States is decreasing from 19% in 1958–1959 to 4.9% today.[16] Based on demographic progression, edentulism will be 2.6% by 2050. With periodontal disease tooth loss 4 times higher in smokers, the continued decreased use of tobacco could drive edentulism yet lower.[17] How can the scope of practice and residency requirements evolve in this setting? As an example, with 97% of today's older Scandinavians already with functionally apposing dentition, the need turns toward maintaining dentition from effects of chronic degenerative diseases and the use of tooth replacement including implants having a more esthetic than functional advantage with regard to societal need has changed the approach to partial edentulism in that setting. A 70-year-old patient with abfraction, degenerative crown lengthening, and so forth in an environment where they would be expected to remain dentate all their life has different treatment planning indications than the patient of the past with failing teeth due to caries and periodontal disease. As safety net institutions, OMS residents are not often given access to older patients with need for esthetic implant reconstruction. Programs must consider individualized solutions to address deficits in clinical case exposure such as these.

To honestly advance clinical education, consideration should be given to discarding the myths regarding competency in the OMS graduate. Among these myths are the contention that *all* residents can or should be competent in all aspects of the specialty, or all aspects of the construct of residencies described above. It is better to believe that all residents will be capable of practicing surgery (with the literal definition of "practicing" intended). A broadly experienced, intelligent, inquisitive, dexterous, and committed new OMS is all that is needed to become a lifelong learner and better surgeon every year they are in practice.

Adapting to the Changing University

Of the 99 accredited US OMS programs, all but 17 civilian programs are sponsored directly by American Universities.[18] These university programs have full-time faculty with university appointments with the full rights and responsibilities associated with university life. OMS residents, staff, and patients also function within the parameters of the university. In contrast, the 17 hospital-sponsored programs mostly have affiliation contracts for faculty in which they are granted full-time geographic appointment, whereas residents, staff, and patients remain the responsibility of the sponsoring hospital.

American universities are in crisis with virtually every aspect of their programs open for revision. They now consider themselves "too expensive, ineffective, and impractical" for today's students.[19] The cost and duration of programs/the value proposition of higher education, the role of faculty, requirements, degree structure, the budget, community engagement, and relevance of programs are in question.

The university environment of today is more intrusive than ever, although sometimes to good effect. Virtually every accreditation standard is governed by the university structure. Internal accreditations, regional accreditation, and university audits are influencing OMS programs today. The medical schools and dental schools are considered critical and, often, contributory components of the budget. Here are some examples, and their impact on programs:

Admissions to residency are subject to oversight regarding the diversity of applicants and enrollees in OMS. The impact of graduates on their communities and states, often scrutinized with objective data, is required. Especially public universities and their boards are vested in those who are being trained in OMS and what are their career paths.

The program culture in surgical residencies is under review. An emphasis on ensuring a humanistic environment for training is now densely entrenched in higher education. This includes the "Hidden Curriculum" in which the activities and career goals of residents is influenced by a subculture not consistent with that of the parent university.

Universities expect the incorporation of adult learning theory into the construct of programs. This includes items such as maintaining attendance records, using active learning methods such as the flipped classroom and experiential learning, objective and reproducible methods of resident assessment, counseling, and remediation.

A scholarly work product is expected of both faculty and residents. Being an academic resource for baccalaureate level programs and to community colleges for clinical rotations, career planning, or research projects with faculty is often demanded.

As a resource, the university offers extensive opportunity for advancing the art of teaching and learning, for interprofessional education opportunities, and for liaisons with other academic units as diverse as business and fine arts.

The medical school remains the most important of all university units for OMS, and it is undergoing changes that require structural changes in both 4-year and 6-year programs. The main ones relate to the loss of basic medical science hours and advancement of clinical experiences into the first and second years of the curriculum. In addition, a greater focus on behavioral sciences, communication skills, and cultural awareness has taken many of the hours formerly devoted to Basic Medical Sciences (BMS). Adapting this into combined OMS MD programs is the critical challenge of many programs today.

Adapting to a Changing Workforce and Practice Model

Physicians, dentists, and OMS are all more likely to be employed by a health system than ever before. Such systems are creating horizontally and vertically integrated delivery models. In medicine, horizontal integration has created large groups with members selecting those components of their practice based on the needs of the system and their individual needs. Vertical integration has created specialized team members in physician assistants, nurses, technicians, and administrators for oral health dental hygiene, dental assisting, and dental therapy. In the vertically integrated health setting where the physician is not the employer role of the doctor is no longer the autocratic head of the team but rather the chief facilitator, and not necessarily the most knowledgeable or technically capable team member.

Adapting to Changing Technology

Exemplified by the acronym MAMAA (Microsoft, Apple, Meta/formerly Facebook Amazon and Alphabet/formerly Google), a changing technology has produced the largest economic, social, and technological entities on the planet. These offer great opportunities for surgical education that will continue to accelerate rapidly. Some examples for now seem destined to transform much of conventional education and practice in the near future, overtaking earlier change and forever altering OMS:

The Metaverse provides opportunity for advanced simulation in surgical practice so

realistic that the learner is globalized and may no longer be only OMS residents. Such cases of surgical simulation learning when developed may be sold as (nonfungible tokens, initially designed to sell artwork or music). Learners across continents can interact with faculty, including surgical experts to participate in virtual surgery. Such learning environments are not democratized but instead will come at considerable economic cost and value to users and generators of surgical education.

The democratized aspect of the Metaverse will be for education that has been commoditized such as anatomy, pathology, or biochemistry. The challenge to achieve clinical medical and dental education in the Metaverse will be overcome but likely at considerable cost. These Metaverse programs, if organized into a Massive Open Online Courses will reduce the unit cost of participating, globalizing, and level accessing to higher education and specifically for access into advanced training.

The concept of grades is being altered by the gamification of didactic and clinical learning in which there are not simply game winners and losers but a pathway for most learners to achieve milestones on the path toward competency. Instead of a grade, criterion-based assessments allow for every trainee to achieve and be recognized for each milestone.

Although the physical capabilities of surgical robotics are quite advanced, enhancement in next generation robots will be via artificial intelligence. A robot that can outperform a human surgeon must be able to outthink the surgeon as well. Defense systems, autonomous drones, and Tesla automobiles are among the systems developing such changes now. Surgery is not far behind.

A New Program Structure: Learning and Practice Communities

The demands of residency education on program directors, faculty, and residents already far exceed the capacity of any program to conform let alone excel in this emerging environment. Programs can no longer be expected to be replicas of one another. Accreditation standards and the expectations of residents and faculty must adapt to the notion that programs will differ substantially in their capacity and desire to embrace all the change that is occurring.

OMS should consider the development of learning and practice communities, which due to technology can offer far greater depth and resources to all programs. The seeds of this change have occurred in admissions, in learning software (such as the Big 10 Sakai educational software platform project), and in online learning. More formal liaisons among OMS programs and with other medical, surgical, and dental education programs will improve education while not exceeding the capacity of OMS educators and the home institution clinical practicum. Such change would further be supported through the development of a universal electronic health record, extension of licensure that supports telemedicine and joint faculty appointments.

The implication of this education model is that it will support improvement in education with greater globalization and access to more advanced subspecialized training. It will additionally support a new practice model of health systems based practice,OMS practicing within the parameters of the policy makers, the payers, and public need. It remains to be seen whether the future of OMS education, enabled by MAMAA, will be a sustainable advantage in OMS education over the simpler times and technologies our faculty know so well.

DISCLOSURE

No commercial or financial interests exist, and no funding sources were used in producing this contribution.

REFERENCES

1. Oral Health in America, executive summary, National Institute of Dental and Craniofacial Research, 2021.

2. Goodall K, Ticku S, Fazio S, et al. Entrustable Professional Activities in Oral Health for Primary Care Provides Based on a Scoping Review. J Dent Educ 2019;83(12):1370–81.

3. Shane D, Wehby G. Affordable Care Act Spillover Gains to Private Dental Coverage for Dependents Widely Shared but Limited Evidence of increased Utilization. J Am Dent Assoc 2020;151(3):182–9.

4. Well TP Vujicic M, Nasseh K. Recent trends in the utilization of dental care in the United States. J Dent Educ 2012;76(8):1020–7.

5. Vujicic M, Buchmueller T, Klein R. Dental care present the highest level of financial barriers, compared to other types of health care services. Health Aff 2014;35(12):2176–82.

6. Arnetz B, Goethe C Reyelts F. Enhancing healthcare efficiency to achieve the quadruple aim: an exploratory study. BMC Res Notes 2020;13:362.

7. Shah M, Gandrakota N, Ali M. Prevalence of and Factors Associated With Nurse Burnout in the US. J Am Med Assoc 2021;4(2):e20336469.

8. Assael L. Dealing in uncertainty. J Oral Maxillofac Surg 2002;60(3).

9. AAMC Careers in Medicine, American Association of Medical Colleges 2022 viewed at aamc.org January, 2022.

10. Competencies for the New General Dentist, American Dental Education Association House of Delegates, April 2, 2008 viewed at adea.org January 2022.

11. Exploring the ACGME Core Competencies,Part 1, New England Journal of Medicine +, June 2016, viewed online at knowledgeplus.nejm.org January 2022.

12. Watson A, LeRoux T, Ogilivie-Harris D, et al. Entrustable Professional Activities in Orthopedics, JBJS 2021;6(2).

13. Carraccio C, Englander R, Gilhooly J, et al. Building a Framework of Entrustable Professional Activities, Supported by Competencies and Milestones, to Bridge the Educational Continuum. Acad Med 2017;92(3):324–30.

14. Miller W, Rollnick S. Motivational interviewing. Third Edition. NY: Guilford Press; 2012.

15. Dye, B, Hsu, KL, Afful J, et al. Vol 37:3 pp200-216

16. Slade GD, Akinkugbe AA. Sanders AE Projections of US edentulism prevalence following 5 decades of decline. J Dent Res 2014;93:959–65.

17. Oral Health in America:advances and Challenges, 2021, National Institute of Dental and Craniofacial Research: Bethesda, MD.

18. Advanced Dental Education Programs in Oral and Maxillofacial Surgery, American Dental Association at Ada.org viewed January 2022.

19.. Kosslyn S, Nelson B, editors. Senator Bob Kerry, building the intentional university: Minerva and the future of higher education. Cambridge, MA: MIT Press; 2017. p. 1–20.

Fellowship Training in Oral and Maxillofacial Surgery
Opportunities and Outcomes

Jonathan W. Shum, MD, DDS, FACS, FRCDC[a],*,
Eric J. Dierks, MD, DMD, FACS, FACD, FRCS(Ed)[b]

KEYWORDS

- Surgical training • Fellowship • Education • Residency • Training • Medical training
- Dental training • Surgical fellowship

KEY POINTS

- Successful applicants tend to have published articles and participated in other scholarly activities. They commonly have a mentor within the subspecialty of their interest.
- Selection of the program is generally based on the breadth of experience available followed by faculty reputation and location.
- Advantages to the successful fellowship graduate include the experience and confidence to provide specialized service and/or more efficient care to patients.
- Enhancements to an academic department with a fellowship program include better mentorship for residents and guidance toward fellowship, as well as an increased level of scholarly.

INTRODUCTION

The author's definition of a surgical fellowship is an additional period of structured surgical training beyond residency that focuses on a narrow component of advanced or unique procedures related to that specialty niche. Surgical fellowships typically last for 1 or 2 years and on completion may qualify the fellow to take an additional board or Certificate of Added Qualification examination. The origins of how one trains to be a surgeon stem from the apprenticeship model and have evolved over the past 100 years to become a structured and monitored process. Currently, formal surgical training begins in residency in which the length of the program depends on the surgical specialty and can vary from program to program. Many fundamental aspects of surgical training were first described by William Halsted, MD, and continue to be an inherent aspect of

training to this day. The Halstedian training model stressed the importance of repetitive clinical encounters and opportunities to participate in patient care under supervision, with increasing complexity and graded responsibility and independence.[1–3] Before the establishment of training standards, the duration of training was dependent on the subjective assessment of a mentor and ranged from 5 to 7 years.[4] In contrast, modern surgical training is defined by a specified period of time, during which the overall time allocated for training includes research, core general surgical rotations, and rotations specific to the surgical specialty. As the curriculum in all residency programs continues to grow to incorporate ever expanding medical knowledge and new techniques, the time available to digest this input has decreased due to duty hour restrictions, evolving guidelines, and time required for documentation. The need for postresidency fellowship training has evolved to meet the

[a] Oral, Head and Neck Oncologic and Reconstructive Surgery Fellowship, Department of Oral and Maxillofacial Surgery, The University of Texas Health Science Center at Houston, 6560 Fannin Street Suite 1900#, Houston, TX 77054, USA; [b] Department of Oral and Maxillofacial Surgery, Oregon and Health Sciences University, Head and Neck Surgical Associates, 1849 NW Kearney, Suite 300, Portland, OR 97209, USA
* Corresponding author.
E-mail address: jonathan.shum@uth.tmc.edu

Oral Maxillofacial Surg Clin N Am 34 (2022) 545–554
https://doi.org/10.1016/j.coms.2022.03.002
1042-3699/22/© 2022 Elsevier Inc. All rights reserved.

interests of the applicants in obtaining supplemental, focused training, as well as to fulfill the manpower needs of hospitals and academic centers.

Medical education reacts to societal trends, as younger generations seek to pursue personal growth through education to achieve one's ambition and potential. In comparison to prior generations, the past 20 years have demonstrated a trend for marriage to occur later in life, in order for individuals to pursue professional objectives.[5,6] These trends, in part, are demonstrated through the increase in the number of residents choosing to pursue fellowship and the number of programs that have formed. The intention of surgical fellowships is to provide a focused experience on a subset of patients that may not have been possible in residency training. Through an intense exposure, and increasing responsibility and autonomy, the fellowship fulfills a Halstedian principle necessary for expertise. The authors explore the motivations of the surgical fellowship applicant and the benefits that are derived from this higher level of accomplishment.

THE APPLICANT

General surgery contains the largest pool of surgical residents, who can pursue a wide variety of fellowships that are available on completion of residency. A review of the current trends on fellowship application demonstrates an increase of subspecialization, with most pursuing fellowship training immediately following completion of their residency.[7,8] In 2011, approximately 45% of surgical residents pursued fellowship climbing to 61.5% in 2019.[9] Surgical residents often make their decision to pursue fellowship by their senior year, as approximately half are undecided in their junior, second postgraduate year[10]; this would suggest the most impressionable time for surgical residents to develop an interest in fellowship would be in their first 2 years of training. The timing to pursue fellowship is similar for OMFS, as residents are immersed into the specialty in their first year, where often times, this can be an eye-opening experience to the opportunities available through the specialty. As the resident progresses in training, the decision to pursue a fellowship is often in the senior year, as positions are often matched 2 years in advance.

APPLICANT DEMOGRAPHICS

The demographic make-up of surgical fellowship applicants are consistent with the current variations that are seen within general surgery residency programs, with men making up 55% to 67% of the applicant pool.[9,10] The female proportion of fellowship applicants has increased over the past 20 years, coincident with the increase in female surgical residents.[10,11] Otolaryngology–head and neck surgery mirrors these proportions with a relative increase in female representation within the specialty at 41.9%; however, proportionately fewer female ENT graduates pursue fellowship training as compared with their male counterparts.[12] The lowest female representation is noted among orthopedic fellowships: 11.9%.[13] Approximately 73.7% of general surgery fellowship applicants were younger than 30 years, with the proportion dropping significantly as it approaches greater than 40 years of age; this suggests that the consideration to pursue fellowship is more common among younger surgical residents when in their second and third postgraduate year of residency.[9] Applicants from university-based programs comprise the largest proportion with 75.6%, with approximately 50% of these applicants having completed residency at a site with a fellowship program.[11]

WHY FELLOWSHIP/POSTRESIDENCY TRAINING

Motivations behind pursuing fellowship show common themes that are present among all surgical subspecialties. Residents obtain exposure to subspecialties while on rotation, and these experiences would determine or confirm interest in the pursuit of fellowship training. As most residents apply from university-based programs that have the respective fellowship program, these opportunities allow for exposure and mentorship. Most surgical residencies provide an assortment of subspecialty rotations that can develop and refine one's interest, but not enough experience to confer proficiency in that area of focus. Limited by restrictions on work hours and elective time, many residents seek fellowships to obtain additional experience.[14] A survey of 2243 otolaryngology residents over a period of 8 years revealed that the most significant reasons to pursue a particular fellowship were desire for additional expertise (34.9%), intellectual appeal (30.4%), and job opportunity enhancement (16.3%). Enhanced compensation and lifestyle/family considerations were the least likely reasons for pursuing a fellowship. In regard to factors that influence the type of fellowship, lifestyle factors and increased compensation were more important factors among men.[9] A study by Reed and colleagues surveyed 2153 general surgery residents on factors that determined their choice of surgical specialty. The 2 most influential factors in the decision process were types of procedures and techniques involved, followed by exposure to a positive role model in the specialty.[10] Applicants for advanced endoscopy fellowship also cite exposure to mentors in the field and demand for the procedures as significant deciding choices for pursuing fellowship,[15] whereas those pursuing hand surgical fellowships cite a driving influence as the variety and breadth of cases as a main reason for choosing this subspecialty.[16]

The same trend to pursue further education and additional experience is seen in dental school graduates where greater than 50% planned to go into some form of advanced dental education immediately after graduation.[17,18] Similarly, mentorship were also top factors in the motivation of dental students to pursue postgraduate pathways and specialties.[19] Considering these trends, the American College of Surgeons (ACS) has incorporated more opportunities for exposure to mentorship. ACS programs such as the surgical specialty roundtable have been implemented to provide exposure and mentorship to medical students and has shown promising results in improving interest.[20] At the resident level, the Young Fellows Association, through the ACS, also offers opportunities for mentorship to residents that may not have had broad access to subspecialties.

SELECTION OF FELLOWSHIP PROGRAM

When a resident has made the decision to pursue specific fellowship training, the next step is to become acquainted with the available fellowships within that domain. Current methods for applicants to gain program information is via the Internet and interpersonal networking. Online match platforms provide centralized program descriptions, contact information, and weblinks to hosted fellowship programs. For example, the San Francisco Match provides applicants a platform to apply to 22 subspecialties, and provides program specific webpages for information and contacts. Other match platforms exist depending on the type of fellowship and may be managed by their respective subspecialty associations, such as the match for OMFS fellowships. The American Association of Craniomaxillofacial Surgery controls the match platform for OMFS and provides access to 15 Head and Neck Oncology/Reconstructive, 9 cleft and craniofacial surgery, and 4 noncategorized fellowship programs. The web site offers basic program descriptions, department Web site weblinks, as well as email addresses to obtain more information and application directions. Unfortunately, most platforms for all subspecialties are considered to be incomplete in detail.[21–25] To enhance the effectiveness of web-based resources, one study attempted to establish standardized criteria that include fellowship education topics and recruitment variables (**Table 1**).[26] As the COVID-19 pandemic has limited travel and social interactions, the content available via the Internet is now essential to compensate for the lack of the traditional methods of information gathering. The pandemic has replaced the classic in person, onsite fellowship interviews with virtual ones, thereby saving the applicants considerable money at the expense of a less intimate appraisal of each program. Sadly, virtual interviews may become a permanent postpandemic change. Common interview topics of discussion are the fellowship curriculum if a formal one exists, operative volume, and

---

Table 1
Pediatric orthopedic surgery fellowship education and recruitment variables

Education	Recruitment
Research	Description
Didactics	Contact information
Rotations	Application process
Case descriptions	SFmatch.org link
Office/clinic time	Salary
Journal club	Current fellows
Call	POSNA.org link
Meetings/conferences	Prior fellow listing
Teaching responsibilities	Prior fellow outcomes
Faculty listing	Video content
Affiliated hospital information	Location description
Quality improvement	Social media links

From Cohen SA, Shea K, Imrie M. An Update on the Accessibility and Quality of Online Information for Pediatric Orthopedic Surgery Fellowships. Cureus. 2021 Sep 7;13(9):e17802.

the variety of surgical cases. Rapport is assessed by both the applicant and the faculty during these interviews as are the relationships and attitudes between the faculty, fellows, and residents. Ultimately, the applicant must process all this and develop a rank list. Studies evaluating selection criteria used by applicants vary slightly between subspecialities. Applicants for hand surgery fellowships value a high-case volume and a broad scope of procedures, whereas advanced endoscopy fellowship applicants identify high procedure volume, program reputation, and geographic location as their most influential factors.[15] Results from a survey of ophthalmic plastic and reconstructive surgery fellowships revealed similar results in which applicants sought out a high volume of procedures/surgeries but also noted that personality of the program director and their impression at the interview were significant in their choice of ranking programs.[27] It is inherent that an individual who is seeking additional training will select for a program with the most clinically rich experience. Program reputation and mentorship are also important factors but are often secondary to the expected surgical experience.

WHAT ARE THE CHARACTERISTICS OF A SUCCESSFUL APPLICANT?

Medical or dental education is a series of gates. The first is a high threshold for the acquisition of critical thinking and knowledge acquisition skills that needs to be met to allow one to pursue professional education; this is the medical or dental admission test. Passing through this gate is only the first of many for those who choose to become highly specialized in a specific field of surgery. At the level of a medical/dental student, board scores, grade point average, and letters of recommendation are assessed before a candidate's entrance into a residency program. Acceptance to fellowship training is often the last gate in this lengthy, multigated sequence. At this level, candidate assessment is usually based on a more subjective evaluation through interview impressions and letters of recommendation, especially those from investigators known to the evaluator. In some specialties such as cardiothoracic surgery, super fellowships are available to those who seek additional training after completion of traditional fellowships. Of those 90 respondents surveyed to had completed this level of training, 34% described obtaining the extra training in preparation for unique cases such as congenital heart deformities. Twenty-four percent reasoned it was required for their future employment.[28] Within OMFS, surgeons with multiple fellowships

are uncommon, but not unheard of. Of the 32 fellows trained at the Portland Fellowship since 1992, 7 have completed another fellowship.

For the level of fellowship, the ability to differentiate the highly motivated applicant can be difficult. A study on the qualities and characteristics of successful applicants sheds some light on what qualities may be advantageous. In a survey of 444 applicants, of which 238 matriculated into pediatric surgical fellowship training, the significant qualities include publications in peer-reviewed journals, more notably in journals with high-impact factors. Alpha Omega Alpha members comprised 32.7% of successful candidates, attending a university-based residency program (84.9%) and/or training at a program with a pediatric surgery fellowship (59.7%).[11] Identical findings were noted in colon and rectal surgery, thoracic, and surgical oncology fellowship matriculation.[29–31] Pediatric surgery fellowships are considered the most competitive. Among successful applicants, the median applicant publication number was reportedly 11, with an impact factor ranging from 2.5 to –9.9.[7] Within the otolaryngology fellowship selection, the performance in an interview and letter of recommendation are the most significant in determining successful candidates.[32,33]

Financial debt and economic considerations are often discussed as potentially significant deterrents to the pursuit of fellowship; however, a review of surveys would suggest this not to be the case. The median burden of financial debt from medical school is reported to be an average of $215,900 in 2018.[34] Although this is a stunning amount, it does not seem to be a deciding factor against fellowship training.[35] Numerous studies reveal that the influence of income and financial compensation is actually a low motivating factor.[9,10,36] The economic impact of pursuing additional training is variable, in that not all subspecialization will lead to greater lifetime total revenue, as compared with a nonfellowship surgeon. Additional years spent in research has been shown to have a negative effect on lifetime total income.[37] In general, academic surgeons in all surgical subspecialities earn less lifetime revenue compared with those in private practice.[38] As previously noted, the primary intention to pursue advanced training is borne out of interest and desire to acquire additional surgical expertise.

APPLICANTS FOR ORAL AND MAXILLOFACIAL SURGERY FELLOWSHIPS

Data on oral and maxillofacial surgery–based fellowships are less defined, and data on these applicants and their selection criteria are limited. The interest and demand for OMFS fellowships are certainly present as witnessed by the proliferating number of fellowship programs listed on the American Academy of Craniomaxillofacial Surgery match platform (www.aacmfsmatch.org). The numbers of programs have increased from 7 in 2013 to 28 in 2021, and the number of candidates applying for fellowship have increased from 8 in 2013 to 31 in 2021 (**Table 2**).[39–42] The motivations to pursue OMFS fellowship and their selection criteria are similar to those seen in other surgical specialties, with the desire to gain additional skills and knowledge being the most influential factors.[43] A 2012 survey examined trends and attitudes regarding head and neck oncologic surgery (HNOS) within American OMFS programs.[44] This study compiled 63 respondents from which 10 programs had a fellowship-trained program director or chair. Although the sample size was small, the investigators concluded that the proportion of programs with an HNOS fellowship-trained program director or chair had more HNOS scholarly activities and had more residents go on to do head and neck oncologic surgical fellowships than do programs that do not have such fellowship-trained faculty.[44] This trend aligns with the results of other subspecialty applicants, as the presence of a mentor in the field is a strong indicator for guiding those interested toward fellowship training. Also, the increased scholarly output and exposure to HNOS places these applicants in an advantageous position on the fellowship match.[44]

THE FELLOWSHIP PROGRAMS

A surgical fellowship program can be established in a variety of settings that include a hospital, an academic institution, or a private practice that can provide the necessary experience to train fellows. All programs have a common goal to train and provide an experience applicable to their focused area of surgery.[45] Along with clinical and didactic benchmarks, almost all programs require scholarly activity, publications, and participation at conferences. The Accreditation Council for Graduate Medical Education (ACGME) sets the standards for US graduate medical education programs and the sponsoring institution.[46] The

Table 2
Listed American Academy of Craniomaxillofacial Surgeons match oral and maxillofacial surgery fellowship programs

Oral/Head and Neck	Craniomaxillofacial	Other
Ascension Macomb-Oakland Hospital	Arnold Palmer Hospital for Children/Orlando Health, Pediatric Craniomaxillofacial Surgery Fellowship Training Program	Houston Methodist Hospital Oral Facial Surgery Institute CMF Trauma and TMJ Fellowship
Boston University Henry M. Goldman School of Dental Medicine	Boston Children's Hospital (BCH)	University of Michigan TMJ and Orthognathic Surgery
John Peter Smith Hospital	Charleston Area Medical Center	University of Toronto Fellowship in Temporomandibular Joint and Orthognathic Surgery
Louisiana State University	Cleft & Craniofacial Center	
Minnesota Head and Neck Surgery	El Paso Cleft and Craniofacial Fellowship	
North Memorial Hospital and Hubert Humphrey Cancer Center	Florida Craniofacial Institute	
Providence Cancer Institute	LSU Health Sciences Center, Shreveport	
University of Alabama at Birmingham	University of Florida (Jacksonville) Pediatric Craniofacial Surgery Fellowship	
University of Florida College of Medicine – Jacksonville	The University of Oklahoma Cleft and Craniofacial Fellowship	
University of Maryland	University of Pittsburgh/UPMC Children's Hospital of Pittsburgh	
University of Miami		
University of Michigan		
University of Tennessee		
UCSF - Fresno/Community Medical Centers		
UT Health Science Center at Houston		

Data from Refs.[40–42]

equivalent governing accreditation organization for US dental education programs is the Commission on Dental Accreditation (CODA). As of 2021, there are 9 CODA-accredited fellowships. Many of these fellowship programs coexist with a residency program and can lead to the misconception that the fellow is using the resources and pirating the experience intended for resident training. The most common concern would be that a decrease in clinical and surgical experience for the residents exists, with a resultant deficiency in their training. This topic has been studied within various specialties, with the upshot being that the presence of a fellow is actually a positive experience.[47] The fellows contribute to the education of residents and in many instances are placed into the role of a junior faculty. In a pediatric surgery study, the fellow demonstrated 87.5% approval from residents, with commentary that described the fellow as very important to their overall training and education. In this instance, the fellow provided didactic teaching sessions and close mentorship in procedures, when compared with faculty.[47] A study evaluating OB GYN resident surgical confidence and case volume revealed a 94% approval rating that the fellow positively affected their learning. No statistically significant difference was found between comfort levels when performing OB GYN surgeries when programs with a fellow were compared with programs without a fellow.[47] A positive relationship was also observed among urology residents and fellows at the University of Toronto. The result of this study defined recommendations that would foster a productive relationship between residents and fellows. These recommendations included the selection of fellows with proficient technical skills, clinical knowledge, and work ethic; this would ensure that the fellow would focus on the specialized training and not on remediation for deficient basic surgical skills. The fellow should ensure that residents are still involved in complex and innovative procedures.[48] Another study compared the resident experience 3 years before and 3 years after the incorporation of a hepatobiliary fellowship and demonstrated positive reviews among the residents and no significant detraction from their surgical experience.[49,50] The recognized benefits of the presence of the fellow far exceeded the perceived fear that the fellow diminishes a resident's learning experience. A fellow also benefits from working with residents, as they develop leadership skills and have the opportunity to become a mentor.

Along with the enhancements in education for residents, the fellow can provide further benefits to the department through increased scholarly activity such as publications and presentations at major conferences. Fellowship programs that demonstrate high academic scholarly activity are often those programs that have the presence of mentors, higher rank on the match list, and train with a large number of residents and fellows.[51,52] A department with many motivated individuals, working within a setting of mentorship, should inherently lead to higher academic output. In numerous studies, applicants who matriculated into fellowships entered with a high number of publications to begin with. The continued effort by the fellow to be academically productive is part of the training process. All ACGME/CODA fellowship programs have program requirements for scholarly activity. These activities can range from publications in peer reviewed journals, quality improvement, population health, and or teaching. A study on the factors that influence academic productivity among oral and maxillofacial surgeons reported that programs with faculty who possess added qualifications such as an MD, MPH, and/or PhD and fellowship completion correlated with higher h-indices and publications.[53] The h-index, is a measure that accounts for both the number and impact of publications. Trends within otolaryngology show that fellowship-trained faculty had a greater number of publications; however, the h-index was not statistically different between fellowship and non–fellowship-trained faculty.[54] These observations would suggest that the applicant enters fellowship motivated, with a high publication count, and will inherently continue this productivity when working with mentors and faculty during their fellowship training years. In fellowships whose duration is 2 years, research time is often protected, and academic output is most productive during the final year.[55] Clinical research experience during fellowship was considered essential, and the opportunity to participate in research activities was used by 71% of vascular surgery fellows who pursued an academic career versus 57% of vascular fellows who went into private practice.[56] These opportunities to pursue scholarly activity can act as a springboard to an academic career and will become significant considerations for promotion and tenure.

DO FELLOWSHIP-TRAINED SURGEONS HAVE BETTER OUTCOMES?

Fellowship training provides a focused experience on specific patient subsets. The increased time and energy spent caring for these patients in a supervised setting should demonstrate benefits in patient outcomes. The fellowship-trained surgeon will be adept in their area of focus but will also have gained collateral experience that can be applied to all aspects of their practice, whether it is familiarity with technological advances, surgical anatomy, and/or techniques. The completion of fellowship provides a groundwork where the "pearls and pitfalls" have been automatically loaded into one's capability as they enter practice. A study comparing fellowship-trained versus non–fellowship-trained surgeons performing orthopedic arthroplasty reported a significant improvement in outcomes among fellowship-trained surgeons. The study reviewed 16,882 total joint arthroplasties and concluded that fellowship-trained surgeons produced shorter mean length of stay, quicker extremity mobilization, and required the use of 25% less opioids in the postoperative phase.[57] Another paper that examined pediatric patients with extremity fractures showed a statistically significant decrease in complication rates among fellowship-trained surgeons.[58] A systematic review of 23 studies demonstrated a positive impact of fellowship training on patient outcomes for laparoscopic surgery. It was noted there were fewer conversions from laparoscopic to open surgery and lower mortality rates for centers with an affiliated fellowship program than centers without. Of note, a comparison of outcomes for senior surgeons versus current fellows showed no differences in rates of mortality, complications, or conversion to open surgery.[59] Furthermore, studies on specialized surgeries ranging from coronary artery bypass graft procedures to radical prostatectomy have shown improved outcomes by fellowship-trained surgeons when matched for years of experience. These outcomes were reported as reduced time from admission to hospital discharge and were associated with lower mortality. Experience has a significant impact on patient outcomes, as a study on surgeon age was associated with decreasing mortality and readmissions.[60–62] There is overwhelming evidence that fellowship training is beneficial for patient outcomes within the host institution. The presence of a fellowship inherently provides a patient care environment of extensive surgical experience within a select group of patients. These studies suggest a compressive effect of fellowship training that packs multiple years of surgical experience into 1 or 2 focused years. Furthermore, another significant factor could also be that fellowship-trained surgeons practice in academic medical centers that have a well-established system for managing specialized surgeries. A multicenter cohort study of academic centers with trauma and surgical critical care fellowship programs demonstrated these improved outcomes with a significant decrease in mortality, length of intensive care unit stay, and hospital stay.[63] The well-known aphorism, "a rising tide lifts all boats," may apply to such centers that are replete with capable, motivated residents, fellows, nurses, and ancillary staff who are well practiced within their specialized skill set.[64]

DISCLOSURE

All authors certify that they have no affiliations with or involvement in any organization or entity with any financial interest or nonfinancial interest in the subject matter or materials discussed in this article.

REFERENCES

1. Osborne MP. William stewart halsted: his life and contributions to surgery. Lancet Oncol 2007;8(3): 256–65.
2. Chung R. Evaluating surgical residents the old school way: Clues to how surgical training works and why. J Surg Educ 2008;65(6):512–3.
3. Kerr B, O'Leary JP. The training of the surgeon: Dr. halsted's greatest legacy. Am Surg 1999;65(11): 1101–2.
4. Dobson J, Walker RM. Barbers and barber-surgeons of london: a history of the barbers' and barber-surgeons companies. Oxford: Blackwell Scientific Publications for the Worshipful Company of Barbers; 1979. p. 171.
5. Cohn D, Passel JS, Wang W, et al. Barely half of U.S. adults are married – a record low 2011. Available at: https://www.pewresearch.org/social-trends/2011/12/14/barely-half-of-u-s-adults-are-married-a-record-low/. Accessed January 8, 2022.
6. Rabin R. Put a ring on it? millennial couples are in no hurry. New York Times 2018. Available from: https://www.nytimes.com/2018/05/29/well/mind/millennials-love-marriage-sex-relationships-dating.html. Accessed January 8, 2022.
7. Yheulon CG, Cole WC, Ernat JJ, et al. Normalized competitive index: analyzing trends in surgical fellowship training over the past decade (2009-2018). J Surg Educ 2020;77(1):74–81.
8. Borman KR, Vick LR, Biester TW, et al. Changing demographics of residents choosing fellowships: long-term data from the american board of surgery. J Am Coll Surg 2008;206(5):782–9.
9. Miller RH, McCrary HC, Gurgel RK. Assessing trends in fellowship training among otolaryngology residents: a national survey study. Otolaryngol Head Neck Surg 2021;165(5):655–61.
10. Reed CE, Vaporciyan AA, Erikson C, et al. Factors dominating choice of surgical specialty. J Am Coll Surg 2010;210(3):319–24.

11. Gupta S, McDonald JD, Wach MM, et al. Qualities and characteristics of applicants associated with successful matriculation to pediatric surgery fellowship training. J Pediatr Surg 2020;55(10):2075–9.

12. Grose E, Chen T, Siu J, et al. National trends in gender diversity among trainees and practicing physicians in otolaryngology-head and neck surgery in canada. JAMA Otolaryngol Head Neck Surg 2022; 148(1):13–9.

13. Oser FJ, Grimsley BM, Swinford AJ, et al. Variety and complexity of surgical exposure, operative autonomy, and program reputation are important factors for orthopaedic sports medicine fellowship applicants. Arthrosc Sports Med Rehabil 2021; 3(3):e855–9.

14. Awan M, Zagales I, McKenney M, et al. ACGME 2011 duty hours restrictions and their effects on surgical residency training and patients outcomes: a systematic review. J Surg Educ 2021;78(6): e35–46.

15. Trindade AJ, Gonzalez S, Tinsley A, et al. Characteristics, goals, and motivations of applicants pursuing a fourth-year advanced endoscopy fellowship. Gastrointest Endosc 2012;76(5):939–44.

16. Harper CM, Johannesdottir F, Rozental TD. Prospective fellows' appraisal of hand surgery fellowships. J Hand Surg Am 2021. S0363-5023(21)00607-00609.

17. Istrate EC, Slapar FJ, Mallarapu M, et al. Dentists of tomorrow 2020: an analysis of the results of the 2020 ADEA survey of U.S. dental school seniors. J Dent Educ 2021;85(3):427–40.

18. Harrison JL, Platia CL, Ferreira L, et al. Factors affecting dental students' postgraduate plans: a multi-site study. J Dent Educ 2021. https://doi.org/ 10.1002/jdd.12792.

19. Nassar U, Fairbanks C, Flores-Mir C, et al. Career plans of graduates of a canadian dental school: Preliminary report of a 5-year survey. J Can Dent Assoc 2016;82:g19.

20. Campwala I, Aranda-Michel E, Watson GA, et al. Impact of a surgical subspecialty roundtable on career perception for preclerkship medical students. J Surg Res 2021;259:493–9.

21. Silvestre J, Vargas CR, Ho O, et al. Evaluation of the content and accessibility of microsurgery fellowship program websites. Microsurgery 2015; 35(7):560–4.

22. Yong TM, Davis ME, Coe MP, et al. Recommendations on the use of virtual interviews in the orthopaedic trauma fellowship match: a survey of applicant and fellowship director perspectives. OTA Int 2021; 4(2):e130.

23. Aryanpour Z, Ananthasekar S, Rajan SS, et al. Evaluation of surgical oncology fellowship websites: are we showing what applicants need to see? Surg Open Sci 2021;7:1–5.

24. Abdou H, St John A, Bafford AC, et al. Assessing content of accredited colon and rectal surgery fellowship websites: is there adequate information for applicants? Am Surg 2021. https://doi.org/10. 1177/00031348211056276.

25. Jain MJ, Chinnakkannu K, Patel DJ, et al. Match for orthopedic fellowship programs in the united states: online accessibility, content, and accreditation comparison between subspecialties and review of alternative resources. Cureus 2021;13(11):e19643.

26. Cohen SA, Shea K, Imrie M. An update on the accessibility and quality of online information for pediatric orthopaedic surgery fellowships. Cureus 2021;13(9):e17802.

27. Shantha JG, Shulman B, Gonzalez M, et al. American society of ophthalmic plastic and reconstructive surgery fellowship survey: Fellows selection criteria for training programs. Ophthalmic Plast Reconstr Surg 2013;29(6):428–30.

28. Bergquist CS, Brescia AA, Watt TMF, et al. Super fellowships among cardiothoracic trainees: prevalence and motivations. Ann Thorac Surg 2021;111(5): 1724–9.

29. Wach MM, Ruff SM, Ayabe RI, et al. An examination of applicants and factors associated with matriculation to complex general surgical oncology fellowship training programs. Ann Surg Oncol 2018;25(12): 3436–42.

30. Shindorf ML, Copeland AR, Gupta S, et al. Evaluation of factors associated with successful matriculation to colon and rectal surgery fellowship. Dis Colon Rectum 2021;64(2):234–40.

31. Drake JA, Diggs LP, Martin SP, et al. Characteristics of matriculants to thoracic surgery residency training programs. Ann Thorac Surg 2021;112(6):2070–5.

32. Johnson J, Stathakios J, Chung MT, et al. Factors important in the selection of a rhinology/skull base surgery fellow: a national survey of fellowship directors. Am J Rhinol Allergy 2021;35(2):234–8.

33. Elsharawi R, Johnson J, Chung MT, et al. Fellow selection protocols in facial plastic surgery: a national survey of facial plastic surgery program directors. Facial Plast Surg Aesthet Med 2020;22(4):309–11.

34. Hanson M. Average medical school debt. educationdata.org Web site. 2021. Available at: https:// educationdata.org/average-medical-school-debt. Accessed January 22, 2022.

35. Jolly P. Medical school tuition and young physicians' indebtedness. Health Aff (Millwood) 2005;24(2): 527–35.

36. Gaskill T, Cook C, Nunley J, et al. The financial impact of orthopaedic fellowship training. J Bone Joint Surg Am 2009;91(7):1814–21.

37. Baimas-George M, Fleischer B, Slakey D, et al. Is it all about the money? not all surgical subspecialization leads to higher lifetime revenue when compared to general surgery. J Surg Educ 2017;74(6):e62–6.

38. Baimas-George M, Fleischer B, Korndorffer JR, et al. The economics of private practice versus academia in surgery. J Surg Educ 2018;75(5):1276–80.

39. American Academy of Craniomaxillofacial Surgeons. AACMFS match results 2021. Available at: https://www.aacmfsmatch.org/match-results. Accessed January 22, 2022.

40. American Academy of Craniomaxillofacial Surgeons. Other-cranio-maxillofacial-surgery. Available at: https://www.aacmfsmatch.org/other-cranio-maxillo facial-surgery. Accessed Jan 8, 2022.

41. American Academy of Craniomaxillofacial Surgeons. Cleft & craniofacial surgery. Available at: https://www.aacmfsmatch.org/cleft-craniofacial. Accessed Jan 8, 2022.

42. American Academy of Craniomaxillofacial Surgeons. Head and neck oncology. Available at: https://www.aacmfsmatch.org/head-neck-oncology. Accessed Jan 8, 2022.

43. Kademani D, Woo B, Ward B, et al. Oral/head and neck oncologic and reconstructive surgery fellowship training programs: transformation of the specialty from 2005 to 2015: Report from the AAOMS committee on maxillofacial oncology and reconstructive surgery. J Oral Maxillofac Surg 2016;74(11):2123–7.

44. Clark PK, Markiewicz MR, Bell RB, et al. Trends and attitudes regarding head and neck oncologic surgery: a survey of united states oral and maxillofacial surgery programs. J Oral Maxillofac Surg 2012;70(3):717–29.

45. Accreditation Council for Graduate Medical Education. The program directors' guide to the common program requirements (fellowship and one-year fellowship). Accreditation Council for Graduate Medical Education; 2020–. https://www.acgme.org/program-directors-and-coordinators/welcome/program-directors-guide-to-the-common-program-requirements/. [Accessed 8 January 2022].

46. Accreditation Council for Graduate Medical Education. The ACGME for residents and fellows. Available at: www.acgme.org Web site. https://www.acgme.org/residents-and-fellows/the-acgme-for-residents-and-fellows/. Accessed January 8, 2022.

47. Backes CH, Reber KM, Trittmann JK, et al. Fellows as teachers: a model to enhance pediatric resident education. Med Educ Online 2011;16. https://doi.org/10.3402/meo.v16i0.7205.

48. Grober ED, Elterman DS, Jewett MA. Fellow or foe: the impact of fellowship training programs on the education of canadian urology residents. Can Urol Assoc J 2008;2(1):33–7.

49. Zyromski NJ, Torbeck L, Canal DF, et al. Incorporating an HPB fellowship does not diminish surgical residents' HPB experience in a high-volume training centre. HPB (Oxford) 2010;12(2):123–8.

50. Altieri MS, Frenkel C, Scriven R, et al. Effect of minimally invasive surgery fellowship on residents' operative experience. Surg Endosc 2017;31(1):107–11.

51. Pearlman SA, Leef KH, Sciscione AC. Factors that affect satisfaction with neonatal-perinatal fellowship training. Am J Perinatol 2004;21(7):371–5.

52. Traylor J, Friedman J, Runge M, et al. Factors that influence applicants pursuing a fellowship in minimally invasive gynecologic surgery. J Minim Invasive Gynecol 2020;27(5):1070–5.

53. Roudnitsky E, Hooker KJ, Darisi RD, et al. Influence of residency training program on pursuit of academic career and academic productivity among oral and maxillofacial surgeons. J Oral Maxillofac Surg 2021. S0278-2391(21)01129-0.

54. Moffatt DC, Ferry AM, Stuart JM, et al. Trends in academic achievement within otolaryngology: Does fellowship training impact research productivity? Am J Rhinol Allergy 2021. https://doi.org/10.1177/19458924211054788.

55. Knuth TE. Trauma fellowship training: the insiders' perspective. J Trauma 1993;35(2):233–40.

56. Henke PK, Kish P, Stanley JC. Relevance of basic laboratory and clinical research activities as part of the vascular surgery fellowship: an assessment by program directors and postfellowship surgeons. J Vasc Surg 2002;36(5):1083–91.

57. Mahure SA, Feng JE, Schwarzkopf RM, et al. The impact of arthroplasty fellowship training on total joint arthroplasty: comparison of peri-operative metrics between fellowship-trained surgeons and non-fellowship-trained surgeons. J Arthroplasty 2020;35(10):2820–4.

58. Livermore AT, Sansone JM, Machurick M, et al. Variables affecting complication rates in type III paediatric supracondylar humerus fractures. J Child Orthop 2021;15(6):546–53.

59. Johnston MJ, Singh P, Pucher PH, et al. Systematic review with meta-analysis of the impact of surgical fellowship training on patient outcomes. Br J Surg 2015;102(10):1156–66.

60. Bilimoria KY, Phillips JD, Rock CE, et al. Effect of surgeon training, specialization, and experience on outcomes for cancer surgery: a systematic review of the literature. Ann Surg Oncol 2009;16(7):1799–808.

61. McAteer JP, LaRiviere CA, Drugas GT, et al. Influence of surgeon experience, hospital volume, and specialty designation on outcomes in pediatric surgery: a systematic review. JAMA Pediatr 2013;167(5):468–75.

62. Satkunasivam R, Klaassen Z, Ravi B, et al. Relation between surgeon age and postoperative outcomes:

A population-based cohort study. CMAJ 2020;
192(15):E385–92.

63. Arbabi S, Jurkovich GJ, Rivara FP, et al. Patient outcomes in academic medical centers: Influence of
fellowship programs and in-house on-call attending surgeon. Arch Surg 2003;138(1):47–51 [discussion: 51].

64. Kennedy JF. Remarks in heber springs, arkansas, at
the dedication of greers ferry dam. the american
presidency project web site.Available at:
presidency.ucsb.edu/documents/remarks-heber-
springs-arkansas-the-dedication-greers-ferry-dam.
Updated 1963. Accessed Jan 28, 2022.

Faculty Development for the Twenty-First Century
Teaching the Teachers

Eric R. Carlson, DMD, MD, EdM[a],*, Eileen McGowan, EdD[b]

KEYWORDS

- Faculty development • Adult learning theory • Andragogy • Mindsets • Emotional intelligence
- Lifelong learning • Holding environments • Deliberately developmental organizations

KEY POINTS

- The primary impetus for individuals assuming faculty positions in undergraduate and graduate medical and dental education programs is largely passion rather than formal training in adult learning theory and education.
- Faculty in undergraduate and graduate medical and dental education programs clearly benefit from structured programs in faculty development. These programs need not be geared to entry-level assistant professors but are of benefit to all faculty regardless of their seniority in their academic departments.
- Although content expertise is essential for a high-performing faculty member, such expertise does not necessarily predict effective teaching methods by faculty.
- Noncognitive characteristics of faculty members, including their mindset, emotional intelligence, and commitment to holding environments and lifelong learning platforms ought to be assessed and enhanced in the best interests of effective teaching and faculty development.

INTRODUCTION AND HISTORY

In the late nineteenth century, US medical schools were little more than a business with instructors profiting from shared tuition generated by large student enrollments. Applicants did not require college preparation for entrance, and curricula were described as trade schools.[1] The 3-year course of study was almost purely didactic, although lectures were poorly prepared by instructors and poorly attended by students. To add to this adverse and inadequate curriculum, the students counterintuitively did not have clinical exposure to patient care. The faculty of these medical schools were considered intellectually competent, presumably as content experts at the time, but their primary intention was to fill the class and graduate doctors.[1] Most students attended private tutoring sessions known as quizzes, expensive teaching sessions at the time to obtain the medical education that they perceived was necessary.

In the fall of 1874, William S. Halsted was one of 550 men to matriculate at the College of Physicians and Surgeons affiliated with Columbia College. Students at this school were assigned a mentor who oversaw the education of several students in each of the 3 classes. Halsted's mentor was Dr. Henry Sands, a surgeon and professor of anatomy, with whom he performed anatomic dissections. With his passion centered on anatomy and surgery, as well as his adequate financial means, Halsted seized numerous opportunities for anatomic dissection by purchasing extra cadavers from which to learn, well beyond the abilities of other students in his class.[1] Halsted clearly benefited by his education and leadership role

a Department of Oral and Maxillofacial Surgery, University of Tennessee Graduate School of Medicine, 1930 Alcoa Highway Suite 335, Knoxville, TN 37920, USA; b Harvard Graduate School of Education, 1165 N Pennsylvania Street, Denver, CO 80203, USA
* Corresponding author.
E-mail address: ecarlson@utmck.edu

Oral Maxillofacial Surg Clin N Am 34 (2022) 555–570
https://doi.org/10.1016/j.coms.2022.02.004

modeling as he became one of the 4 founding fathers of Johns Hopkins Hospital in 1889 along with Dr. William Welch in pathology, Dr. Howard Kelly in obstetrics and gynecology, and Dr. William Osler in medicine.

Like Halsted, Osler was critical of medical education and commented on its unfortunate condition as part of his address to the Medical and Chirurgical Faculty of the State of Maryland in April of 1889, just prior to assuming his position as chief of the Department of Medicine at Johns Hopkins Hospital:

> It makes one's blood boil to think that there are sent out year after year scores of men, called doctors, who have never attended a case of labour, and are utterly ignorant of the ordinary everyday diseases which they may be called upon to treat: men who may never have seen the inside of a hospital ward and who would not know Scarpa's space from the sole of a foot. Yet, gentlemen, this disgraceful condition which some school men have the audacity to ask you to perpetuate; to continue to entrust interests so sacred to hands so unworthy. Is it to be wondered, considering this shocking laxity, that there is a widespread distrust in the public of professional education and that quacks, charlatans, and imposters possess the land?

The inadequacy of medical education exposed by Osler resulted in the realization of guilt of the entire medical establishment, and the system had to be changed.

In 1907, Abraham Flexner, an American educator, was charged by the Carnegie Foundation to scrutinize the structure of medical education in North America. Flexner identified numerous unacceptable qualities of medical education, primarily related to its proprietary nature. In June 1910, his legendary report entitled *Medical Education in the United States and Canada – A Report to the Carnegie Foundation for the Advancement of Teaching* called for educational reform with prerequisites including completion of high school, at least 2 years of university, 4 years of medical school in a university setting that involved 2 years of basic science and 2 years of clinical clerkships, followed by postgraduate training in the form of specialty residency education.[2] The treatise consists of 14 chapters in 181 pages of his research findings and conclusions, primarily focused on the disparity between the proper basis and actual basis of medical education at the time, as well as Flexner's suggestions for the course of medical study over 4 years.

Recommendations for reconstruction of medical education were included in the first part of the lengthy document. Finally, part 2 of Flexner's thesis centered on the medical schools located in 39 states and Canada. The report contains an intriguing and thought-provoking introduction provided by Henry Pritchett, the president of the Carnegie Foundation, and the fifth president of Massachusetts Institute of Technology from 1900 to 1906, who aptly pointed out that institutions of higher learning at that time were sensitive to external criticism. This notwithstanding, Pritchett indicated that colleges and universities adhered to the belief that they were private organizations such that the public was privy to knowledge of their inner workings as the organization chose to communicate. Further, some institutions reported by the Flexner report challenged the right of an outside agency to collect and distribute details of their medical schools. He indicated that the foundation's conviction was that all colleges and universities, both public and private, represented public service corporations, such that the public was permitted to know the facts associated with the financial and educational aspects of their administration and development. Pritchett opined the following concepts regarding the Flexner Report:

1. For the 25 years prior to the Report, there had been an over-production of uneducated and ill-trained medical practitioners.
2. The existence of uneducated and ill-trained medical practitioners was directly due to the presence of an excessive number of commercial schools.
3. The quintessential feature of a medical school was a profitable business.

In the late nineteenth century, dentistry was a nascent profession that was not highly respected by the medical profession.[3] Dr. James Garretson, professor of oral surgery at the Philadelphia Dental College, indicated in 1875 that he was "most decidedly in favor of the abolishment of the degree DDS. One degree in medicine is enough; the greater covers the lesser and includes it."[3] Therein, during this time, dental education could justifiably be criticized as being substandard, as well. Formal dental education in the United States began in 1840 with the establishment of the Baltimore College of Dental Surgery. Other dental schools slowly began to emerge, gradually displacing the traditional preceptorship method of training for dentistry. The period of the late 1800s saw a surge in the number of dental colleges in the United States. These schools were largely proprietary in nature, as they were not affiliated with major universities, were private, and were of a commercial nature and, usually established to benefit their owners, not unlike the early medical schools.[4] In 1881, the American Medical Association adopted oral surgery as a specialty of medicine.

As the trend toward affiliation of dental schools with universities gained impetus at the beginning of the twentieth century, and with the establishment of the Dental Educational Council of America, the trend continued. Finally, the Carnegie Foundation for the Advancement of Teaching formed a committee, under the direction of Dr. William J. Gies, to study the entire system of dental education in the United States. Out of this landmark study came the stout recommendation that all dental schools become affiliated with major universities. After that study, in the early 1930s, the last proprietary school was abolished. This article traces the histories of dental schools, past and present, in the United States.

The Flexner Report of 1910 set the stage for the creation of requisite qualities of medical faculty in general and the structure of medical education. Specifically, content expertise can be perceived to have been emphasized as essential to the educational process, yet without any regard for its effectiveness and calibration in the learning process, in large part to the lack of understanding of adult learning theory, the application of Socratic teaching in medical education, and coregulated learning in undergraduate and graduate medical education. This notwithstanding, Flexner's principles of reconstruction of US medical schools called for these schools to be university departments, located in large cities, only 1 school being assigned to a single town, and arrangements made to provide the required infrastructure within each state. Finally, the postgraduate school was a concept of great interest to Flexner. The postgraduate school, akin to a medical residency, was established to provide education not accomplished by the medical school, thereby serving as an "undergraduate repair shop." Flexner commented on 13 postgraduate schools of the time, including the Postgraduate and Polyclinic of New York and the Polyclinic of Philadelphia. According to Flexner, those facilities commanded extensive dispensary services and hospital clinics. He stated that the teaching at these sites was immediately practical to be scientifically stimulating as it had the "air of handicraft, rather than science." The courses were disconnected, however, and the faculties were huge and unorganized.

More than 100 years following the publication of the Flexner report, the professional roles and expectations of medical and dental educators of the twenty-first century are evolving in response to the transformation of medicine and dentistry, as well as the art and science of teaching. In fact, the professional identities of faculty as teachers provides a profound influence on the academic productivity of these individuals.[5] To foster and enhance the identity of an academic physician will likely pay dividends in terms of that physician's academic productivity. Indeed, the effective teacher, more than anyone else, has the ability to favorably affect eternity.[6] Unfortunately, although their identities as revenue-generating clinicians and grant-producing researchers are supported by academic medical centers, their identities as teachers do not receive a similar degree of acclaim and recognition. Therein, the perception of the lack of appreciation of academic faculty by health systems leads to dissatisfaction regarding one's teaching role and possible abandonment of an academic career.[7] Further, even when systematic support of the identity of academic physicians exists, self-imposed pressure to produce clinically may often result in a lack of academic productivity on the part of academic physicians. Numerous moving parts exist in the faculty development arena, therefore, and change is at the core of all anticipated progress. The context of teaching the teachers is complex and exemplifies the realization that faculty recruitment and retention represent inseparable yet distinct disciplines. Their unifying element, however, is change that provides individual and collective development of faculty. It is anticipated that effective faculty development through teaching the teachers initiatives will instill enhanced identity in academic physicians, with this identity supplanting the physician's perception of relative lack of worth by health systems. Stated differently, the magnitude of an academic physician's identity as a teacher should translate to that physician's perception of worth and relevance. Unequivocally, creating an element of change in that physician's teaching presence, with a resultant sustainable academic identity, is the means to an end in this regard. One must establish a platform of faculty development with a construct of change within individuals and their academic medical centers.

THE CONCEPT OF CHANGE

In October 2016, Dr. Edward Verrier delivered the John H. Gibbon Jr. Lecture at the American College of Surgeons Clinical Congress in Washington, DC.[6] He pointed out that the basis for surgical education had changed minimally in the 106 years since the publication of the Flexner Report. He reported that the personal computer had replaced the printing press during this time, and that international society had progressed from the telephone to the Internet. Transformations had occurred in the practice of medicine due to a logarithmic growth in knowledge, regulations in practice, surgical efficiency, and the publication of transparent outcomes data. This notwithstanding, Verrier indicated that surgical education had not substantially changed in its style of teaching during this 106-year period of time.[6] Therein, among others, he recommended several considerations for faculty with change as the overarching principle:

1. The cultivation of growth mindsets by faculty
2. Recruitment of residents with grit, not merely for perceived talent based on their background and biased letters of recommendation and the results of short applicant interviews
3. Making faculty development a priority in academic medical centers for all faculty while formally creating programs that permit teaching the teachers rather than assuming that master clinicians are master teachers
4. Promoting and formally recognizing academic productivity through incentivization
5. Improving deliberate practice in surgery while leveraging simulation, rehearsal, and coaching
6. Critically reviewing didactic teaching sessions while moving from teacher-centric positivism to learner-centric, case-based, experiential learning with flipped classrooms
7. Developing nontechnical, noncognitive, and nontraditional curricula where leadership, emotional intelligence, coping with loss, professionalism, and formative feedback are collectively emphasized.
8. Improving the educational expectations in the operating room where learner and educator preparation is required; move from the checklist huddle to an educational huddle with briefs and debriefs while insisting on proficiency rather than mere competency
9. Ceasing the undervaluation of teaching and mentorship, while placing greater emphasis on coaching and understanding the difference between each discipline
10. Being responsible earlier adopters and agents of change

THE NEUROSCIENTIFIC BASIS FOR CHANGE

The term plasticity was initially applied to the central nervous system, and specifically to the brain in 1890 by William James and later referred to as neuroplasticity by Jerzy Konorski in 1948.[8] These terms reference the changes that occur in brain function and structure throughout life. Neuroplasticity reflects the exemplary capability of the brain to adapt and change and suggests that complex physiologic changes in the brain result from interactions between the organism and its environment. Such a dynamic process allows the brain to adapt to different experiences and to learn. Neuroplasticity is observed on numerous scales, with adaptive behavior, learning, and memory existing at the top of the neuroplasticity hierarchy with synaptic communications between the brain's 86 billion neurons forming the basis for these changes.[8] In fact, in the 1890s, Adolf Meyer, the chairman of psychiatry at Johns Hopkins University from 1910 to 1941, noted that the concept of neuroplasticity was supported by the observation that neurons were not physically connected.[9]

Holtmaat and Caroni[10] point out that learning and memory are associated with the development of neuronal assemblies, a group of neurons that are collectively recruited because of their synaptic connections, most commonly resulting from the learning process. These neurons maintain strengthened synapses to ensure collective and simultaneous activity, although these neurons might not be physically close to one another. Neuronal assemblies are thought to represent the smallest physical counterparts of representations in the brain such that neurons pertaining to a specific assembly are located within numerous regions of the brain. In memory and learning, neuronal assemblies likely form, undergo modification, and dynamically dissolve.[10] Neuronal assemblies that account for memories would therefore be identified during the learning process. These assemblies would provide access to information that had been learned upon appropriate recall cues and would then provide for further learning. The important operational criteria that define neuronal memory assemblies include their selective reactivation being sufficient to produce behaviorally effective memory recall and their inactivation preventing memory recall. Assemblies of neurons recruited during learning are likely related to the ensembles of neurons encoding the corresponding memory. A neuronal ensemble is considered a population of neurons involved in a specific computation. The term is commonly used within systems and neuroscience to describe a neural network with a specific function. Carillo-Reid and Yuste[11] define neuronal ensemble as a group of neurons repeatedly firing synchronously. They point out that the interaction of numerous neuronal ensembles at a given time and the sequential activation of distinct neuronal ensembles could endow neural circuits with increased computational capacity. Such computational capacity likely translates to effective change and learning.

For some time, it was believed that neuroplasticity peaked at a young age and then gradually diminished as people aged. The expression, "You can't teach an old dog new tricks," exemplifies this misunderstanding. The evidence in support of the concept of lifelong neuroplasticity has been noted by greater sophistication of medical imaging of brain structure and function.[12] Deliberate practice, for example, leads to improved and refined performance on motor and other tasks and this dynamic behavior process is associated with altered brain activity that occurs similarly in young and older subjects.[12] Aside from functional changes in the brain, deliberate practice also results in structural changes such as alterations in gray and white matter that are recruited during task performance. Pauwels and colleagues[12] point out that the gold standard to produce neuroplasticity is through the intensive practice of new tasks and to organize training in a way to maximize the learning and retention of new skills. These authors indicated that the emergence of neuroplasticity requires the creation of a sufficiently challenging practice context for learners. For example, rather than performing tasks in a sequential fashion, one after the other that is less challenging, one can apply a more demanding practice regime such that learners switch tasks from trial to trial during practice that is more challenging. The latter regime has led to the apparent paradox that reduced performance levels are obtained during the training phase, but more durable long-term retention and memory formation of the skill are ultimately observed, resulting from more profound intertask information-processing strategies. This concept is referred to as contextual interference (CI). Although contextual interference produces a more complex learning environment, it has been demonstrated that older adults can cope under these circumstances, as can younger adults, and that this technique benefits durable skill retention.[12] The intertask information processing strategies resulting in contextual interference in a teaching the teachers framework involve the concepts of mindsets, emotional intelligence, and lifelong learning, among other elements of change. It is these tasks and their inherent contextual interference that provide beneficial change to leaders in undergraduate and graduate medical and dental education in the context of effective faculty development through teaching the teachers.

FACULTY DEVELOPMENT STRATEGIES – TEACHING THE TEACHERS
Mindsets

Dr. Carol Dweck, the Lewis and Virginia Eaton Endowed Professor of Psychology at Stanford University, published her seminal work in 2006 entitled *Mindset: The New Psychology of Success*.[13] In the 2016 update of her work, Dweck outlined her theories related to fixed and growth mindsets. The fixed mindset is possessed by those individuals who incorrectly believe that they are born with a fixed amount of intelligence, basic ability, and talent (**Table 1**). These individuals commonly avoid challenges and resist any possibility of failure, thereby eliminating their opportunities for learning, growth, and self-improvement. By contrast, the growth mindset designates those individuals who recognize that change exhibited by practice, willing effort, and perseverance will result in unlimited opportunities for growth and self-improvement (see **Table 1**). The growth mindset is fundamentally based on the belief of individuals recognizing the value of, and the inherent ability to change while developing personally and professionally. These agents of change accept challenges with great enthusiasm and are not stymied by the potential for failure or fleeting humiliation, but rather grow in response to its inevitability. The wholly opposed growth and fixed mindsets are noted to exist simultaneously in all people, and our successes and failures are dictated by whether we knowingly or unknowingly choose to conduct our personal and professional lives through the lens of a fixed or growth mindset.[14] Our ability to gravitate toward a growth mindset as change agents requires that we fully recognize the presence of our fixed mindset thoughts and actions. Stated differently, the view that individuals adopt for themselves profoundly affects how individuals lead their lives.[13] Faculty can deliberately change their mindset to further their professional development, and faculty development frameworks should assess mindsets and teach the teacher to the path of a growth mindset. In the context of our foundation of faculty development, Brock and Hundley[14] discussed the primary circumstances when a mindset can be identified, including the individual encountering challenges and obstacles, their execution of effort, their response to criticism, and their reaction to the success of others (see **Table 1**).

The attributes of a growth mindset faculty member have been discussed from which a framework for faculty development can be contextualized. These attributes include flexibility, having high expectations, being communicative, building strong

Table 1
Qualities and defining features of the fixed versus growth mindset

Fixed Mindset	Growth Mindset
Belief that ability and talent are fixed or limited and that improvement in an area is not possible if one does not exhibit natural talent in that area; effort is required for those who cannot otherwise succeed.	Belief that success is a direct result of positive-thinking effort put forth, rather than one's natural ability or talent
Tendency to avoid challenges to avoid failure or appearing incompetent; failure is unacceptable and feared	Tendency to approach challenges without fear of failure; failure is inevitable in professional development and anticipated without fear
Tendency to give up after encountering an obstacle	Willingness to try a new strategy when encountering an obstacle
Tendency to blame others or underlying circumstances for failure	Tendency to view failures and mistakes as stepping stones to more successful outcomes
Rarely identifies lack of effort as the cause of failure	Ability to readily identify the link between effort and achievement
Tendency to shut down in the face of mistakes	Tendency to be energized by failure as an opportunity to grow and overcome a problem
Views mistakes as an embarrassment, not a learning opportunity	Demonstrates understanding that mistakes are a part of the learning process
Tendency to view feedback as criticism and/or personal attack	Tendency to seek feedback as productive criticism and as a necessary ingredient for growth
Threatened and envious by the success of others	Cognizant of the ability to learn from the success of others
Entity theory (implicit) of intelligence: intellect is unchangeable.	Incremental theory (implicit) of intelligence: intellect can be grown or developed over time
Academic mindset (entity theory) is to look good.	Academic mindset (entity theory) is to learn
Non-resilient.	Resilient
Avoid conflict management.	Meet adversity directly without fear for conflict

Adapted from Brock A, Hundley H. In other words. Phrases for growth mindset: a teacher's guide to empowering students through effective praise and feedback. Ulysses Press; 2018: 3-4.

relationships, being process-oriented, valuing mistakes, being empathetic, possessing positive interdependence, and being equitable.[14] The authors acknowledge the essential nature of tractability in the education of students and residents as adult learners, thereby not exposing them to antiquated, impractical, and educationally immaterial and nonevidence-based concepts and techniques. The authors believe in teaching students and residents how they learn rather than expecting them to learn the way teachers teach.[15] They recognize that effective faculty development begins with high expectations of every student and resident and that those expectations are modeled "through body language, verbal communication, positive reinforcement, and constructive feedback."[14] The authors ascribe to effective communication and interaction with students and residents whereby they do not feel they are being pimped for information based on an academic hierarchy, but rather that they are participating interactively in coregulated learning for the simultaneous advancement of their education and proper patient care.[15] The authors advocate for the building of strong personal and professional relationships in the development of faculty, relationships that are based on emotional intelligence. They recognize the value of being process-oriented and understand that effective education is often more about the process than the outcome.

The authors propose that faculty must innovate, and that self-improvement and innovation are inherently subject to failure that should be occasionally anticipated and must not be viewed personally. Failure unequivocally represents a progression in the journey of effective faculty development and faculty learning. The authors recognize that empathy is an important element of emotional intelligence and one that can be taught through change. They emphasize the importance of positive interdependence whereby a community of coregulated learners consists of faculty, students, and residents working toward common goals with favorable patient outcomes. Educators in undergraduate and graduate medical and dental education should teach through their experiential learning and constructive development rather than solely based on positivism, a noninteractive form of teaching. Finally, the authors appreciate the value of distributing resources to student and resident learners in an equitable fashion. Faculty members who do not want to change likely believe that they are entitled, that they need not change, but rather that the world around them should change. Moreover, these fixed-mindset individuals embrace the status quo, believing that their lives are acceptable, and their teaching styles are sufficient and legacy issues, in that they have always done things that way. The fixed mindsets of these individuals are preventing faculty development, at the core of which is reticence to change.

Yeager and Dweck[16] presented research data in 2021 that concluded more favorable student achievement when students believe or are instructed on the basis that intellectual abilities can be cultivated rather than representing a quality that is fixed. These authors indicated that psychological interventions that change the mindsets of students are successful, and educators should encourage such mindset changes. Significant in this psychology are the implicit theories of students. Yeager and Dweck defined implicit theories as "core assumptions about the malleability of personal qualities."[16] They explained that these theories are implicit, because they are uncommonly made explicit, and theoretic, because "they create a framework for making predictions and judging the meaning of events in one's world."[16] Additionally, Yeager and Dweck explained that students may fluctuate in their implicit theories from a relatively fixed entity theory of intelligence to a more flexible incremental theory of intelligence. The academic mindset of a student with the entity theory of intelligence is to appear intelligent, yet a tendency to despair exists when challenged. These students have a relatively high value of effort because they feel that they lack the ability, and academic performance suffers during times of adversity. The academic mindset of a student with an incremental theory of intelligence is to learn and to work harder when challenged. These students have a relatively lower value of effort and their academic performance increases during times of adversity. The authors' contextualization of faculty development is to inculcate the ability and desire within faculty to stimulate the incremental theory of intelligence in students and residents.[15]

The prototypical framework of faculty development is encouraged through change toward more uniform application of growth mindsets and through the recognition of identity as teachers. Therein, contemporary faculty development activities include initiatives that support the technical skills and adaptive challenges of faculty members.[15,17] In their final analysis, the authors recognize that faculty members with growth mindsets are learners, whereas faculty members with fixed mindsets are nonlearners.[16] Establishing faculty development programs that emphasize growth mindsets and identity as teachers represents a more favorable enhancement of professional development than those that merely address the technical and adaptive elements of faculty development. To realize excellence in both teaching and learning, faculty members must be taught to embrace their identities as teachers through adoption of growth mindsets, and this identity must be supported by their academic medical centers through transformative faculty development programs. Faculty exhibiting shifts from fixed mindsets to growth mindsets will effectively educate and maintain learning environments through which students and residents will receive the prime clinical and didactic education they expect, require, and deserve.

Emotional Intelligence

Emotional intelligence is described as a form of social intelligence that permits the thoughtful oversight of the emotions of oneself and that of others, while permitting the comparing and contrasting of these emotions and directing one's thinking and actions accordingly.[18] Goleman[19] comprehensively outlined the 5 components of emotional intelligence, including self-awareness, self-regulation, motivation, empathy, and social skill (**Table 2**). Johnson[20] defined emotional intelligence as various noncognitive attributes and competencies that assist individuals to cope with the demands and stressors of their environment. Davies and colleagues[21] defined emotional intelligence as an attribute consisting of 4

Table 2
The definition and hallmarks of the 5 components of emotional intelligence

	Definition	Hallmarks
Self-awareness	The ability to recognize and understand moods, emotions, and drives, as well as their effect on others	Self-confidence Realistic self-assessment Self-deprecating sense of humor
Self-regulation	The ability to control or redirect disruptive impulses and moods The propensity to suspend judgment – to think before acting	Trustworthiness and integrity Comfort with ambiguity Openness to change
Motivation	A passion to work for reasons that go beyond money or status A propensity to pursue goals with energy and persistence	Strong drive to achieve Optimism, even in the face of failures Organization commitment
Empathy	The ability to understand the emotional makeup of other people Skill in treating people according to their emotional reactions	Expertise in building and retaining talent Cross-cultural sensitivity Service to clients and customers
Social skill	Proficiency in managing relationships and building networks An ability to find common ground and build rapport	Effectiveness in leading change Persuasiveness Expertise in building and leading teams

From Goleman D. What makes a leader? In: HBR's 10 must reads on emotional intelligence. Harvard Business Review Press; 2015:6; with permission.

characteristics: appraisal and expression of emotion in oneself, appraisal and recognition of emotion in others, regulation of emotion in oneself, and the use of emotion to facilitate performance. Individuals with high emotional intelligence can use, comprehend, and manage emotions effectively to their benefit and to the benefit of others. Emotional intelligence is integral to the Socratic method of teaching and represents an effective strategy for change in undergraduate and graduate medical and dental education. Therein, the change in a teacher's emotional intelligence serves as an essential construct in faculty development and should be considered in teaching the teachers frameworks.

The utility of emotional intelligence in undergraduate and graduate medical education learning environments serves 2 purposes. First, resident physicians learn more effectively when their teaching is performed with compassion, consistent with Socratic teaching.[22] Secondly, the execution of emotional intelligence by faculty should translate to effective modeling for residents who in turn will develop their own style of emotional

intelligence and transfer such expression to their patient interactions. In assessing the use of emotional intelligence strategies in undergraduate and graduate medical and dental education settings, 4 questions become paramount[20,21,23]:

1. What is emotional intelligence, and how can it be measured?
2. What is the relevance of emotional intelligence to a communication skills educator, and how can its focus assist in the development of emotional intelligence in learners?
3. How can emotional intelligence contribute to the selection and development of students and residents?
4. What methodological issues are associated with incorporating emotional intelligence-based education into postgraduate curricula?

A retrospectively viewed noncompassionate teaching style represented a rite of passage for junior academic faculty and residents of years past. Unkind criticism of residents who failed to answer questions correctly with the subsequent execution of public shame led by faculty and senior residents was often the norm rather than the exception. The hopeful anticipation for a surgical intern was an attending surgeon or surgical faculty member who did not ascribe to such practices. Under these circumstances, learning was historically more effective, and residents gravitated toward these attending physicians who frequently did not possess faculty appointments in academic medical centers and who paradoxically provided more practical education to trainees than the formal and hierarchical academic faculty, much to the dismay of these faculty members. This observation ultimately gave way to a subsequent generation of faculty members who possess emotional intelligence.

One additional component of emotional intelligence exhibited by faculty in graduate medical education settings is related to leadership style. The distinction of transformative versus transactional leadership styles has been observed to have a significant influence on team performance.[24] Transactional leaders are task focused, typified by conditional reward with precise assignment of responsibility for performance targets and the rewards for their achievement, and management by exception with focus of attention on mistakes/failures. Although such goal focused leadership may achieve task performance and the realization of favorable outcomes, it may also predispose the team to fatigue.[24] By contrast, transformational leaders are characterized by idealized influence with a focus on the collective mission, inspirational motivation, intellectual stimulation, and consideration of individual needs.[24] Transformational leaders not only recognize the requirements of team members, they also conscientiously strive to develop these team members. In doing so, they encourage others to evolve and perform according to expectations. Transformational leaders motivate performance and discretionary behaviors that are not directly assigned to a single team member, but which sustain the culture and environment necessary to predict effective and efficient collective team function. Transformational leaders in surgery are those with emotional intelligence.[24]

Johnson[20] determined what is known about emotional intelligence and the role it plays in relationships and its essential nature within health care and medical education. Specifically, she assessed the value of emotional intelligence in health care settings and the ways in which this skill can be incorporated in medical education. A direct correlation between medical education and emotional intelligence competencies was concluded in her review. When addressing the ability to teach emotional intelligence, numerous issues must be considered. It is first necessary to establish a likely rationale for the process required to learn emotional intelligence. Secondly, one must consider the effectiveness of evidence related to attempts to teach emotional intelligence. Finally, the diverse factors related to successful implementation of emotional intelligence programs must be investigated, because educational environments are complex and dynamic.[20]

The concept of emotional intelligence as a learned skill allows for training in specific competencies that can be directly applied to educators in undergraduate and graduate medical and dental education fields. When emotional intelligence is conceptualized as a skill that can be taught, learned, and changed, it may be used to address the interaction of the resident and faculty member to improve the educational process. Therein, emotional intelligence training should be a priority of graduate medical education faculty development platforms to enhance personal/professional relationships.

Holding Environments

The concept of an effective holding environment in educational settings may be extrapolated from the prior discussion of emotional intelligence. First described by pediatrician and psychoanalyst, Dr. D.W. Winnicott and later elaborated by developmental psychologist, Dr. Robert Kegan, the concept may be applied to various types of supportive structures across the lifetime, but it presents particular advantages to medical and dental education. At its core, a holding environment offers a balanced distribution of emotional support and compassionate learner challenges across time. Stated differently, a holding environment sustains empathetic collaboration exhibited by emotional intelligence. Within a medical teaching setting, faculty development at all levels can be advanced through guidance, support, administrative and academic nourishment, and other elements of an environment that provide opportunities for personal growth in one's career.

The creation of a holding environment ensures individual and collective professional growth and serves 3 important functions. First, the environment recognizes and confirms the identity of the individual in terms of how he or she currently understands role and function without urgently pushing for change. In other words, this space must accept individuals for who they are and how they are making meaning in their faculty position. Individual value is validated. Second, the environment must challenge, stretch, or encourage the faculty member to let go and grow beyond current understandings. This challenge element might take the form of difficult discussions, challenging assignments, or suggestions for growth. Finally, the holding environment must remain in place as the faculty member grows in new ways so that supportive relationships can be reformed as required to permit continued growth.[25] Drago-Severson[25] considers a holding environment to be a context in which adults feel well held psychologically, supported and challenged developmentally, understood in terms of how they make sense of their work, and accepted and honored for who they are. Stated differently, holding environments are learning contexts in which adults feel relevant, heard, and comfortable taking the risks they require to grow academically and professionally. Although the concepts of confirmation, challenge, and continuity may appear conventional, a deeper dive into this concept leads one to understand that these functions depend on the developmental level of the participants and must be approached accordingly. For instance, a beginning student or resident may feel threatened by too much challenge without considerable support, whereas a senior faculty member may relish significant questioning of practice while not needing or appreciating constant praise and reinforcement. Thus, this is a sophisticated concept that requires high levels of emotional intelligence to use effectively.

There are clear benefits to fostering a holding environment in undergraduate and graduate medical and dental education. The first benefit occurs on an individual level and includes interpersonal exchanges between individual residents and faculty, which offer advice, direction, evaluation, or a collegial conversation to support that resident's personal growth. Again, this is a highly individualized experience. Given what is known about the reciprocal nature of true mentoring relationships, it not only affords the student or resident the opportunity to become more independent and self-authorizing, but the teaching faculty may also experience growth through generativity or the passing of wisdom to the next generation. The second benefit can occur at an institutional level in which the organization itself experiences a positive change in culture. The balanced orientation of confirmation, challenge, and continuity ideally permeates groups of students, residents, and faculty and becomes manifest in the approach of academic department chairs and residency program directors at all levels. Evidence of this cultural shift has been documented in various professional settings in the work of Kegan and Lahey entitled *An Everyone Culture: Becoming a Deliberately Developmental Organization*.[26]

What is especially encouraging about this concept is that it applies to people across the lifespan, signaling a lifelong learning philosophy, as will be discussed. In a deliberately developmental setting, therefore, both senior faculty and nascent students are offered the opportunity to grow and change. With a high level of emotional intelligence, holding environments in undergraduate and graduate medical and dental education settings incorporate a high level of psychological safety that enhances education.[27]

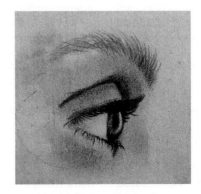

SUBJECT

That which we unquestionably assume to be true, something with which we are fused, and therefore something we are unable to reflect or question. Figuratively speaking, we *cannot* see this knowledge.

OBJECT

Something that is separate or distinct from oneself, and something that we can organize and potentially change. Figuratively speaking, we *can* see this knowledge.

Fig. 1. The subject and object characteristics of adult learning theory.

Lifelong Learning

Learning is a discipline of one's personal and professional development that exists in numerous constructs, and a discipline that occurs at different times during one's lifetime. The education of children and adolescents is highly structured in terms of curriculum, while the education of adults is more typically diverse, multifactorial, and subject to self-direction. As described by Malcolm Knowles, adult learning can be distinguished from learning by children by self-concept, experience, readiness to learn, orientation to learning, and motivation to learn, in which adult learning theory is more advanced and individualized than that of children.[28] Lifelong learning is vastly different from adult education in that the latter represents opportunities for formal learning in one's adult life without additional specification. The challenge for lifelong learning, by contrast, is to reconsider the impact of learning and education with the intention of changing the learner's mindset.[28] Specifically, lifelong learning involves the acquisition and application of new knowledge and skills in the framework of self-direction. Therein, a subject to object shift occurs in educational goals and objectives (**Fig. 1**). As occurs in regimented and requisite educational platforms, learners are subject to their education in that these individuals unquestionably assume material to be true and not able to be questioned. Such educational materials are often subjected to rote memorization for success on examinations. Kindergarten-12th grade (K-12) curricula are prime examples in that limited choice exists in the selection of coursework. By contrast, adult learning often permits the participant to be object to their education. Under these circumstances, the adult learner is specifically able to reflect on educational material with its organization and change. Moreover, the subject to object shift that occurs in the lifelong learner is beneficial to the integration of work and learning, thereby permitting the development of insight into the context of one's work on meaningful professional issues.[29] The recipients of lifelong learning, therefore, become agents of change in terms of their personal and professional lives and often that of those around them.

Robert Kegan's constructive development theory of adult learning emphasizes the organizational structure of an adult's learning process rather than the contents of that educational system. The stages of adult development and adult learning theory specify the elements that structure one's thinking, feeling, social relations, and learning or how the individual thinks, feels, and knows rather than what the individual thinks,

feels, and knows. The socializing mind or third order of consciousness, also referred to as the socializing mind, is possessed by people who are aligned with, and identify with an ideal, a group, or a relationship that is more meaningful than their own impulses, desires, or needs (**Fig. 2**). In terms of lifelong learning, the third order of consciousness is subject to the educational structure and paradigms of teachers, curricula, and organizations (**Fig. 3**). If mistakes are made, responsibility for them is usually positioned outside of the self. The allegiance of these individuals to the expert opinions of their teachers is sacrosanct and not questioned. Therein, self-direction is relatively absent in these individuals such that the socializing mind is limited in terms of the ability to change as a result of engagement in lifelong learning and its benefits in terms of faculty development. According to Carlson,[28] it can be argued that lifelong learners ascribe to a higher order of consciousness, specifically self-authoring, or self-transforming minds.

The fourth order of consciousness, also known as the self-authoring mind, exhibits a more integrative self that is mentally more complex than the third order of consciousness. Fourth order individuals are object to abstract thinking, and they represent an authority that is responsible for designating its own belief system, including its self-direction. These individuals are internally motivated, although they value the actions and opinions of others and determine what is best for themselves. In terms of lifelong learning, self-authoring learners accept knowledge as a framework for interpreting and analyzing experience with the recognition that knowledge develops from internal curiosity and a deep sense of responsibility for their learning capacity, quintessential characteristics of lifelong learners (see **Fig. 3**). The purpose of all education for self-authoring minds is to become something other than what they currently are, to expand their horizons, and to serve as agents of personal and organizational change.

The fifth order of consciousness, also known as the self-transforming mind, is demonstrated by individuals whose thinking is dialectical, indicative of an increasing awareness of, and orientation to paradox, contradiction, and oppositeness. In terms of lifelong learning, fifth order individuals see themselves as temporary, incomplete, and perpetually in the state of reinvention (see **Fig. 3**). Rather than accepting themselves as constructed at any given time, self-transforming minds identify with their evolution. Although the self-authoring mind identifies with the preservation of limits and boundaries as a method of distinguishing and defining the self, the self-transforming mind

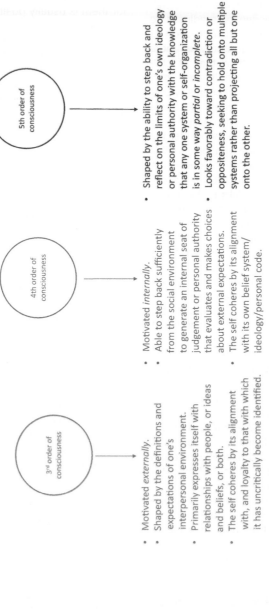

3rd order of consciousness

- Motivated *externally*.
- Shaped by the definitions and expectations of one's interpersonal environment.
- Primarily expresses itself with relationships with people, or ideas and beliefs, or both.
- The self coheres by its alignment with, and loyalty to that with which it has uncritically become identified.

4th order of consciousness

- Motivated *internally*.
- Able to step back sufficiently from the social environment to generate an internal seat of judgement or personal authority that evaluates and makes choices about external expectations.
- The self coheres by its alignment with its own belief system/ideology/personal code.

5th order of consciousness

- Shaped by the ability to step back and reflect on the limits of one's own ideology or personal authority with the knowledge that any one system or self-organization is in some way *partial or incomplete*.
- Looks favorably toward contradiction or oppositeness, seeking to hold onto multiple systems rather than projecting all but one onto the other.

Fig. 2. The 3 orders of consciousness with increasingly greater mental complexity.

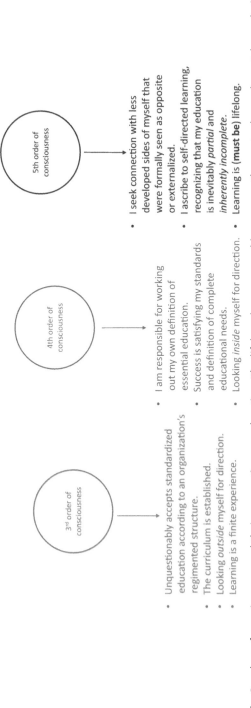

3rd order of consciousness

- Unquestionably accepts standardized education according to an organization's regimented structure.
- The curriculum is established.
- Looking *outside* myself for direction.
- Learning is a finite experience.

4th order of consciousness

- I am responsible for working out my own definition of essential education.
- Success is satisfying my standards and definition of complete educational needs.
- Looking *inside* myself for direction.

5th order of consciousness

- I seek connection with less developed sides of myself that were formally seen as opposite or externalized.
- I ascribe to self-directed learning, recognizing that my education is inevitably *partial* and *inherently incomplete.*
- Learning is (**must be**) lifelong.

Fig. 3. The 3 orders of consciousness and their perspectives on education. The lifelong learner arguably possesses the most advanced mental complexity.

demonstrates tentativeness and reticence to accept achievement as anything other than temporary and preliminary. Individuals who align with the self-transforming mind and who reject the limitations of the self-authoring mind do so with the intention of addressing their partial and incomplete states. In many respects, the enthusiasm for, and the execution of lifelong learning is indicative of the transition of the self-authoring mind to the self-transforming mind.

The self-authoring and self-transforming minds are fertile ground for effective and durable faculty development. These individuals, although different, are nonetheless aligned in terms of their need to contribute something of importance to society, often with the intention of associating with something bigger than themselves. To this end, the subject-object interview serves as a lens for faculty development. This interview serves to assess the motivation for lifelong learning, its execution, and the objective plan to obtain additional learning. The faculty member should share with the subject-object interviewer the what, so what, and now what associated with their desire for lifelong learning. The what addresses the perceived need for additional education by the faculty member. What could represent a self-directed interest, but additional information from the subject-object interview is required to state such. The so what ascertains the motivation associated with lifelong learning. The now what serves the purpose of identifying the application of the additional education for the faculty member's lifelong learning plan. If the motivation for lifelong learning is perceived by the interviewer to be externally driven, the learner represents a socializing mind (see **Fig. 3**). The establishment of internal motivation is required to establish at least the fourth order of consciousness in the learner. The identification of a plan established through introspection as a primary influence rather than motivation provided by an employer or family member leads the interviewer to suggest a mental complexity at least that of self-authorship (see **Fig. 3**). The faculty member's quest for lifelong learning to address incompleteness in his or her ideology or personal authority is most suggestive of the self-transforming mind (see **Fig. 3**).

Continuing medical education (CME) is required of all practicing clinicians to support ongoing licensure in one's field and hopefully stimulating that individual's learning trajectory. Nonetheless, CME in the form of weeklong or weekend courses does not satisfy the definition of lifelong learning. McAdams and McNally[30] provided a comparison of continuing medical education and lifelong learning. They explained that physician motivation plays a

significant role in lifelong learning. Specifically, there are sources of autonomous motivation and controlled motivation in the self-determination theory of motivation. Autonomous motivation occurs through intrinsic motivating factors and provides a longer-lasting, positive form of motivation. Controlled motivation occurs through extrinsic sources of motivation including rewards and avoidance of punishment. With this type of motivation, outcomes are shorter lasting and less favorable. Because it is known that lifelong learning is more associated with autonomous motivation, developers of curricula must understand these motivations with the intention of creating deep learning environments for the lifelong learner. Talati[31] argues that CME is not a form of lifelong learning, but rather learning across the lifespan (LAL). LAL is usually spaced and not continuous of any major goal. The gaps in education result in principles and ingrained concepts that are lost. Talati[31] indicates that the most useful lifelong learning for physicians is that which is continuous, has no endpoint, no preformed curriculum, and no assessment other than reflective metacognitive activity. This notwithstanding, the lifelong learner would have a well-defined source for learning in society and well-defined direction with clear benefit to society. Talati[31] stated that lifelong learning is internally driven in contrast to the externally driven learning that is required to satisfy professional needs in the realm of recertification and job transitions.

In considering the essential nature of lifelong learning in faculty development platforms, the authors offer the rules of Erren and colleagues,[32] consistent with the principles of Hamming regarding lifelong learning:

1. Cultivate lifelong learning as a style of thinking that concentrates on fundamental principles rather than on facts.
2. Structure learning to ride the information tsunami rather than drown in it.
3. Focus on the future, but do not ignore the past.
4. Look for the personal angle.
5. Learn from the successes of others.
6. Use trial and error to find the style of learning that suits you.
7. No matter how much advice one gets and how much talent one possesses, it is still the individual who must do the learning and put in the time.
8. Have a vision to enable general direction.
9. Make life count: struggle for excellence.

These rules resonate with the self-directed, individualized, and highly thought-provoking nature of lifelong learning, and provide invaluable advice to faculty members and their advisors in achieving goals for such learning.

SUMMARY

Accrediting and professional organizations within organized medicine and dentistry have embraced the essential nature of faculty development in the twenty-first century. These organizations include the Accreditation Council on Graduate Medical Education (ACGME), the Commission on Dental Accreditation (CODA), the American Dental Education Association (ADEA), and the American College of Surgeons (ACS).[33] Common to the faculty development strategies of these organizations are examples of compliance including attendance and national meetings, understanding of relevant aspects of teaching methodology, curriculum design and development, and development of new clinical skills. The faculty member largely depends on his or her motivation to demonstrate compliance. Simpson and colleagues[34] point out that in 2025, the role of the faculty developer will result in faculty navigating complex learner assessment data, and to achieve acceptable performance targets utilizing shared mobile technology. To this end, Simpson and colleagues[34] identify new roles for faculty educators in 2025 as

1. Content curator
2. Technology adapter
3. Learner-centered navigator and professional coach
4. Learning environment designer, engineer, architect, and implementer
5. Clinician role model

Moving forward, it is important for all faculty in undergraduate and graduate medical and dental education programs to be knowledgeable about content with the ability to accurately quote the literature. Faculty should effectively teach content while also guiding learners to achieve performance targets. But, mastering content knowledge and meeting performance targets is not sufficient. Given knowledge of growth mindsets and lifelong learning, one must reconceptualize medical and dental education as a lifelong pursuit. This orientation will allow the profession to keep pace with a rapidly changing world of technology and research. Teaching faculty must adapt technology in teaching methods to teach students and residents the way in which they learn rather than expecting them to learn the way one teaches. Faculty members must create effective learning strategies that support personalized learning and developmental growth. A focus on emotional intelligence offers the path to a deeper understanding of faculty, residents, and patients and provides an atmosphere of psychological safety. Creating an environment that is deliberately developmental means promoting surroundings that confirm and challenge medical and dental professionals while they change and learn new ways of existing. And finally, teaching faculty should serve as effective role models for students and residents with the hope of creating the next generation of teachers in undergraduate and graduate medical and dental education.

DISCLOSURE

Dr E.R. Carlson receives book royalties from Wiley Blackwell, Elsevier, and Quintessence Publishing.

REFERENCES

1. Imber G. Genius on the edge. The bizarre double life of Dr. William Stewart Halsted. New York: Kaplan Publishing; 2011. p. 21–2.
2. Flexner A. Medical education in the United States and Canada. A report to the Carnegie Foundation for the advancement of teaching. New York: The Carnegie Foundation for the Advancement of Teaching; 1910. p. 1–346.
3. Punjabi AP, Haug RH. The development of the dual-degree controversy in oral and maxillofacial surgery. J Oral Maxillofac Surg 1990;48:612–6.
4. Schulein TM. A chronology of dental education in the United States. J Hist Dent 2004;52:97–108.
5. Steinert Y, O'Sullivan PS, Irby DM. Strengthening teachers' professional identities through faculty development. Acad Med 2019;94:963–8.
6. Verrier ED. The elite athlete, the master surgeon. J Am Coll Surg 2017;224:225–35.
7. Davis DA, Rayburn WF, Smith GA. Continuing professional development for faculty: an elephant in the house of academic medicine or the key to future success. Acad Med 2017;92:1078–81.
8. Gulyaeva NV. Molecular mechanisms of neuroplasticity: an expanding universe. Biochemistry (Moscow) 2017;82:237–42.
9. Lamb S. Neuroplasticity: a century-old idea championed by Adolf Meyer. CMAJ 2019;191:E1359–61.
10. Holtmaat A, Caroni P. Functional and structural underpinnings of neuronal assembly formation in learning. Nat Neurosci 2016;19:1553–62.
11.. Carillo-Reid L, Yuste R. What is a neuronal ensemble? Oxford Research Encyclopedia, Neuroscience. Oxford, England: Oxford University Press USA; 2020. p. 1–23.
12. Pauwels L, Chalavi S, Swinnen SP. Aging and brain plasticity. Aging 2018;10:1789–90.

13. Dweck CS, Mindset. The new psychology of success. New York: Random House; 2006.

14. Brock A, Hundley H. In other words. Phrases for growth mindset. A teacher's guide to empowering students through effective praise and feedback. Berkeley, CA: Ulysses Press; 2018.

15. Carlson ER, Tannyhill RJ. The growth mindset. A contextualization of faculty development. J Oral Maxillofac Surg 2020;78:7–9.

16. Yeager DS, Dweck CS. Mindsets that promote resilience: when students believe that personal characteristics can be developed. Educ Psychol 2012;47:302–14.

17. Heifetz RA. Leadership without easy answers. Cambridge: Harvard University Press; 1994. p. 73–6.

18. Salovey P, Mayer J. Emotional intelligence. Imagin Cogn Pers 1990;185–211.

19. Goleman D. What makes a leader? In: On Emotional intelligence. Boston (MA): Harvard Business Review Press; 2015. p. 6.

20. Johnson DR. Emotional intelligence as a crucial component to medical education. Int J Med Educ 2015;6:179–83.

21. Davies M, Stankov L, Roberts RD. Emotional intelligence: in search of an elusive construct. J Pers Soc Psychol 1998;75:989–1015.

22. Carlson ER, Tannyhill RJ. A foundational framework for andragogy in oral and maxillofacial surgery II: interactive andragogies. J Oral Maxillofac Surg 2019;77:1101–2.

23. Carlson ER, Tannyhill RJ. A foundational framework for andragogy in oral and maxillofacial surgery III. Emotional intelligence. J Oral Maxillofac Surg 2019;77:1324–6.

24. Hu YY, Parker SH, Lipsitz SR, et al. Surgeons' leadership styles and team behavior in the operating room. J Am Coll Surg 2016;222:41–51.

25. Drago-Severson E. Helping educators grow. Strategies and practices for leadership development. Cambridge, MA: Harvard Education Press; 2012. p. 47.

26. Kegan R, Lahey LL. An everyone culture. Becoming a deliberately developmental organization. Cambridge: Harvard Business Review Press; 2016.

27. Nembhard IM, Edmondson AC. Psychological safety: a foundation for speaking up, collaboration, and experimentation in organizations. In: Spreitzer GM, Cameron KS, editors. The Oxford handbook of positive organizational scholarship. Oxford, England: Oxford University Press; 2015. p. 1–26.

28. Carlson ER. Lifelong learning: a higher order of consciousness and a construct for faculty development. J Oral Maxillofac Surg 2019;77:1967.e1–8.

29. Carlson ER. Lifelong learning and professional development. J Oral Maxillofac Surg 2016;74:875–6.

30. McAdams CD, McNally MM. Continuing medical education and lifelong learning. Surg Clin North Am 2021;101:703–15.

31. Talati JJ. Lifelong learning: established concepts and evolving values. Arab J Urol 2014;12:86–95.

32. Erren TC, Slanger TE, Grob JV, et al. Ten simple rules for lifelong learning, according to Hamming. Plos Comput Biol 2015;11:e1004020.

33. Carlson ER. Academic relative value units: a proposal for faculty development in oral and maxillofacial surgery. J Oral Maxillofac Surg 2021;79:36.e1–13.

34. Simpson D, Marcdante K, Souza KH. The power of peers: faculty development for medical educators of the future. J Grad Med Educ 2019;11:509–12.

Mentoring, Coaching and Role-Modeling in Surgical Education

James R. Hupp, DMD, MD, JD, MBA[a],*,
Leslie R. Halpern, MD, DDS, PhD, MPH, FICD[b]

KEYWORDS

- Mentor • Mentee • Coach • Teacher • Role-model • Two-way mentorship

KEY POINTS

- The legacy of mentorship has undergone a transformation from the traditional apprenticeship model to a more *"collegial paradigm"* using innovative strategies tailored to the mentee's individual aspirations and challenges.
- An effective mentor will enhance the mentee's productivity and ability to achieve success; however, mentors must be compatible on numerous levels including an alignment of values to ensure the long-term success of the mentorship.
- A variety of mentoring strategies can be beneficial within the surgical training environment, facilitated by learning in the operating room and when rounding, hours spent caring for patients, and time spent mastering surgical strategies and technology, all of which the mentee must achieve for professional growth.
- Coaching, teaching, and mentorship should encourage the self-reflection that is critical for a surgical resident to reach their goals and become a successful practitioner.

INTRODUCTION

Qualifying for and getting accepted into an oral-maxillofacial surgery residency was a challenging endeavor for most of us, and continues to be so for the current generation of dental students. Furthermore, once in residency, the challenges continue, and in some ways heighten. Fortunately, residency training is a shared experience, with similarly aged cohorts available to offer emotional support and with whom to commiserate. Coresidents are also a valuable source of learning throughout one's residency years. However, although residents give each other a substantial amount of information and guidance, they too are still on their journey to becoming an oral-maxillofacial surgeon (OMS); therefore, their ability to share knowledge and wisdom based on years of experience are understandably limited.

A decade ago, Assael stated: *"Mentoring is the single most powerful tool to the learning and practice of surgery"*[1] An editorial by Hupp in the Journal of Oral and Maxillofacial Surgery suggests;" *two-way mentoring"* so that both parties are accountable with respect to their roles and responsibilities.[2] By doing so, the mentee not only receives the positive impact from his/her mentor(s), but more importantly, attains the surgical knowledge to benefit the surgical care of their patients and future legacy of surgeons who will follow. Residency faculty and others serve to complement and greatly enhance the education and training resources necessary for each resident to become an OMS. However, ideally, simply finishing a residency and becoming certified should only be considered the first stage of an OMS's career development. The ultimate goal should be for

[a] Elson S. Floyd College of Medicine, Washington State University, Spokane, WA, USA; [b] Oral and Maxillofacial Surgery, University of Utah, School of Dentistry, Salt Lake City, UT, USA
* Corresponding author.
E-mail address: James.hupp@wsu.edu

Oral Maxillofacial Surg Clin N Am 34 (2022) 571–576
https://doi.org/10.1016/j.coms.2022.03.007

each resident trainee to reach their full career, and even life, potential. This is where other forms of career guidance come into play.

This article discusses how the mentoring of oral-maxillofacial surgery residents can better optimize their chances to have a meaningful and impactful career (meaningful; being of value to one's self and impactful; being of value to others). Other forms of guidance, such as coaching and role-modeling, will also be compared and contrasted with mentoring; all 3 may overlap and often complement each other. It is important to delineate the meanings of the terms mentoring, coaching, and role-modeling as used in this article. There can be some overlap, but important distinctions exist in the dynamics between the one providing guidance and the recipient of the guidance.

HISTORICAL PERSPECTIVE OF MENTORING

The history of the concept of mentoring as it relates to career development in general, and surgical training, in particular, is useful to consider. Mentoring, as a term, seems to have arisen from Homer's "The Odyssey." Odysseus wanted someone to watch over and guide his young son, Telemachus, during a long 20-year absence to travel and fight wars. He selected a friend named Mentor for this duty. However, as the story goes, Mentor was not up to the task and Telemachus became insecure and indecisive. However, the goddess Athena was watching over Odysseus and intervened to assist Telemachus by assuming the form of Mentor and providing Telemachus with more appropriate guidance.[3]

In the 19th century, the beginnings of a form of surgical "mentoring" arose. It was referred to as a "preceptorship;" however, it was not mentoring as we consider it now, rather it was more similar to an apprenticeship under someone older and more experienced. Some surgeons used their preceptees more like servants than younger colleagues, individuals not ready to be independent even though fully trained. Although Theodor Billroth is credited as the first true surgical mentor of his time, William Halstead was the creator of a formal approach to surgical mentorship we now follow. Halstead's emphasis on the use of scientific evidence to support decision-making closely resembles what today's surgeons use to practice evidence-based medicine.[4]

Throughout the 20th century, mentorship was transmitted into the homes of many who dreamed of becoming surgeons. Numerous television shows depicted practicing surgeons as infallible mentors to their younger colleagues and residents, that is, *Ben Casey* and *Dr Kildare*. Programs such as *Marcus Welby, MD*, provided an "idealistic" view of how doctors provide care, with limited racial diversity of the actors chosen to portray health care providers, including physicians. Doctors were stereotypically males while nurses were female. As the 21st century unfolded, more contemporary television including shows, such as *Gray's Anatomy*, displayed a more modern approach to mentorship in medicine and the demands that both mentors and mentees face in providing patient care. Newer medical shows include more gender diversity/equality among doctors and increased numbers of doctor-educators from wider variety of races and ethnicities. This mirrors the rapidly increasing diversity of surgical trainees in the 21st century, as well as the changing demographics of the patient population being served. These changes have brought a shift in surgical mentorship allowing for more innovative approaches and greater opportunities to enhance the career and personal success of all residents being mentored.[5–7]

CONTEMPORARY PARADIGM OF MENTORING RESIDENTS

The basic residency certification process always includes educators who have the responsibility to educate and train residents (education, in this case, implying the teaching of basic knowledge; training being the teaching of clinical skills relevant to becoming an OMS). The educators can serve in other fashions, but this may or may not occur in each program or for every trainee in a program. Therefore, others outside of the OMS attending staff may serve to support resident career guidance. The educators, faculty, and in some cases, administrative staff, engaging with residents daily who work to prepare residents to be qualified for oral-maxillofacial surgery certification are most often referred to as the resident's teachers (see later in discussion).

THE MENTOR AND MENTEE

The medical literature abounds with articles on the subject of mentorship; however, it is clear there is no one widely accepted definition. Healy and colleagues in their review of surgical mentors and role models, use the Committee on Postgraduate Medical Dental Education in the United Kingdom's definition of mentor as a "process whereby an experienced, highly regarded, empathetic person (the mentor) guides another (usually younger) individual (the mentee) in the development and reexamination of their own ideas, learning and professional development."[8] The mentor should teach by example, encouraging, motivating, and promoting the independence of the mentee and rejoicing in their success.[9] On the other hand, mentors should exert caution as their actions can be detrimental. Examples might be failing to include the mentee in an article for publication with which the mentee assisted or acting inappropriately with operating room staff in front of the mentee. Negative mentoring, as such, can result in lasting negative behavior by the mentee that negates any positive mentoring that has taken place.[10–13]

Mentoring is not simply cheerleading. Mentors carry the responsibility to provide their mentee sage advice, including accurate feedback and a balanced view of what the mentee needs to do to succeed. This may require giving strong constructive criticism if the mentee is not living up to their true potential or have behavioral or personality issues that are interfering with their career development. Straight talk from a respected mentor is usually a powerful motivator.

Mentor

The ideal mentor both exhibits and encourages positive characteristics such as how to best serve one's patients, make sound decisions, work in a collaborative fashion with colleagues including other types of health care professionals, and how to conduct oneself in their life in general. This ideal may be difficult to achieve, as the practice of surgery has become more complex and there is more emphasis by mentees in the areas of work–life balance and personal development.

Geraci and colleagues describe 3 parameters of an effective mentor: 1) exhibiting a degree of seniority, reputation, and experience likely to improve the mentee's potential for success, 2) the mentor and mentee must be compatible on numerous levels (have the "right chemistry") and alignment of values to help ensure the long-term success of their relationship, and 3) the mentor should not be in a supervisory role over the mentee with the inherent conflicts of interests.[6] The dynamics of effective mentoring include active-listening, emotional support when needed and regular encouragement. In addition, mentors should be prepared to learn from and experience professional growth with their mentees, sometimes referred to as two-way mentoring.[2]

Mentee

Historically, the mentee was known as a protégé (favorite), derived from the French verb, protégée (to protect). It is important to note that mentees also have responsibilities, as they are important to ensuring the achievement of the goals of the relationship.[14] Mutual respect and regular communication between mentor and mentee are foremost. It is best for the mentee to be proactive from the onset, seeking out a potential mentor, or preferably, mentors. The selection is commonly based on the potential mentor's expertise, academic standing, professional characteristics, and/or availability. The mentee should seek input about potential mentors from their faculty and peers and do so as early as possible during their surgical training to gain the maximum benefits.[5,15–17] Mentees can seek mentors for various aspects of their training. For example, if conducting research is part of their plans, a mentor with research expertise is preferable. If an academic career is planned, a successful academician makes sense, whereas if a private practice career is more likely, having a mentor successfully practicing in that arena is more appropriate. If a mentee has a particular area of surgery for which they hope to focus on once certified, someone with a practice focus in that area would be wise to approach. Women residents will commonly want to find a female surgeon to serve as at least one of their mentors, recognizing the special challenging still facing women residents and surgeons. Similarly, residents from historically underrepresented ethnicities and races should seek out a mentor or mentors with a similar set of life challenges. Ultimately, the mentee will find it advantageous to seek different mentors to address distinct aspects of their professional and personal lives.[18–20]

The mentee must make clear their own expectations for the relationship and how they hope the mentor will help craft and assess progress toward the mentee's goals in both formative and summative metrics. Three key objectives needed for success are clearly defining: (1) the anticipated goals of the mentorship, (2) the role of each of the participants, and (3) the structure of the mentorship program. Finally, mentorships are not always of value to a mentee. For one, the hoped-for chemistry may not pan out at all or over time. A mentor's or even the mentee's limited availability can hinder/compromise the success of the relationship. As time passes, the mentee may find their need for continuing with a particular mentor wane. On the other hand, the mentor may become frustrated if their advice to their mentee is resisted or ignored. In any case, if either the mentee or mentor determines the mentorship has run its useful course, a straightforward professional discussion should ensure ending the formal mentorship with appropriate gratitude shown and a door left open to renew the relationship if desired by both parties.

ROLE MODELS, COACHES, TEACHERS

A lack of consensus to define what a mentor exemplifies has led to crafting other definitions of protégé' support.[14,21] Mentors can serve as role models, coaches, and/or teachers, but role models, coaches, and teachers are not automatically mentors.[22] (**Table 1**) Mentors, teachers, and coaches are typically aware they are serving in those capacities, whereas a role model is frequently unaware of their impact on others. If a mentor plans to serve in the capacity of a coach and/or teacher, it is wise to prospectively set some boundaries so as to not mislead the mentee as to what aspects of their surgical or personal development goals are being met by the mentor. Sometimes surgical residents have some confusion over the terminology or role being played by individuals they encounter during training. Some residents may call someone their mentor even though they are, in reality, serving more as a role model. It is important for residents to make it clear to anyone they consider a "mentor" that the supposed mentor is aware of the relationship and is willing and prepared to serve in that capacity.

Role models

A role model is predicated on the demonstration of "how to be a successful, high-quality academic physician through example alone and may be passive on the part of the senior academician."[11] It encompasses someone whose professional behaviors are mirrored by the mentee with respect to qualities they would like to have, as well as positions that they would lie to reach. A role model is someone who demonstrates some aspect or aspects of themselves that others seek to emulate. In a residency program, is predicated on the demonstration of "how to be a successful, high-quality, academic physician through example alone and may be passive on the part of the senior academician."[5] Role-modeling encompasses educators whose professional behaviors or bearing mirror the surgical resident's aspirations of qualities they would like to acquire, as well as perhaps, positions they would like to attain. In most places, the surgical role model has evolved from a traditional demanding individual to a trusted team leader with a strong reputation, professional leadership style, and excellent communication skills. Studies have found that a student's choice of surgery as a career is based on the presence of positive surgical role models. Residents exposed to these positive attributes often express how the impact of words, actions, and attitudes become a part of their behavior, perpetuated by the resident, thereby becoming a positive role model for

their junior colleagues. Although most mentors are role models, most role models are not mentors. The differences relate to the amount of ongoing personal interaction, with nonmentor role models taking no part in providing regular career or personal guidance to those viewing them as their role model.

Coach

Coaching is used to provide a specific level of knowledge or aid in achieving a defined goal. It is directed by a task master (coach) who concentrates on this goal. It is most commonly witnessed in sports, whereby, say, a baseball pitching coach helps an individual improve the speed and accuracy of their pitches. The qualities of coaching include aspects of mentoring, as well as teaching, and can form an intricate part in the training of surgeons as coaching focuses on growing and improving surgical skills. In surgical residency, this approach is often conducted during surgery or as a debriefing after the operative case involving reflection, constructive feedback, and emphasizing positive performance.[22,23] The structural approach of coaching is usually individualized to suit each trainee's particular needs and level of training. A coach has the potential to help a surgical trainee change his/her unconscious deficiencies to conscious ones, as well as encouraging greater awareness of conscious abilities to help maximize the resident's potential.

There are 2 types of coaches; expert and peer surgical coaching. The expert coach is one who provides instructional approaches for the learner to self-assess and accept constructive feedback when learning a new skill set.[5] Technological adjuncts include; that is, overhead cameras to help refine the surgeon's coarse and fine movements, as well as a series of didactic and simulation training modules with a set of defined outcomes through procedural training.[10,15] Peer surgical coaching is bidirectional with surgeons that are at a similar level of experience and share approaches as a nonjudgmental partnership.[10,16] The coach must have the appropriate knowledge and expertise and encourage their "coachee" to be bidirectional in ideas and expertise. Both the coach and their "coachee" gained value with respect to their skillset to align roles and cultivate mutual trust as surgical colleagues.[16] Both expert and peer coaching have both advantages and disadvantages. Residency training affords limited time, concerns about reputation, and a loss of control, all of which impedes effective coaching. Several solutions include increased self-awareness and efficiency, select a private location

Table 1
Characteristics of effective mentors, teachers and coaches

Mentors	Teachers	Coaches
Knowledgeable	Knowledgeable	Knowledgeable
Sincere	Expert communication skills	Strong interpersonal skills
Available	Approachable	Cultivates mutual trust
Stimulate enthusiasm	Passion for their subject area	Facilitates learner-directed
Trustworthy	Good technical skills	Highly respected
Flexible	Adapted to different learning styles	Adapts approach to individual learner goals
Good listening skills	Good listening skills	Active listener
Challenges the mentee	Set clear objectives	Recognizes the learner's abilities and experience
Evaluates their own effectiveness	Strong rapport with learners	Nonjudgmental
Track record with other mentees	Organized	

Modified from Lin J, Reddy RM. Teaching, Mentorship, and Coaching in Surgical Education. Thorac Surg Clin. 2019 Aug;29(3):311-320.

to improve and select individualized goals to increase self-directed learning. Taken together the coaching relationship serves as a partnership for helping the learner help themselves.

Teacher

Teaching is similar to coaching, but usually on a broader scale. It commonly involves taking a body of knowledge on a topic and helping the student learn that body of knowledge. This can include helping the student become able to use various learning skills effectively so the student can, in essence, learn how to teach themselves. The evolution of teaching in both medicine and surgery has included innovative approaches that require independent study, simulation exercises, research projects, and episodic and longitudinal patient care. The teacher–resident relationship in surgical training encompasses both didactic and technical skills components. Contemporary teachers now approach learning in a wide variety of venues and encourage their students to be self-directed learners, using the teacher as a resource rather than the totality of what needs to be learned in the resident's surgical discipline.[5] A resident's mentor can be a teacher, but a resident's mentor is not required to help teach the mentee surgery.[22–24]

SUMMARY

Mentors, coaches, and teachers need to understand generational differences in values, life goals, and motivating influences to be effective in working with contemporary surgical residents. The current generation of residents is often characterized as being self-centered and demanding. However, in reality, they generally have laudable values including a desire to serve others less fortunate than themselves and give back to society. They also value life balance (aka work–life balance). This generation usually prefers to work in teams rather than alone and a major demand they have is to be taught using methods that differ from the conventional Socratic method or lecture format.[1,2] They are willing to question authority and see less value in memorization, knowing that most facts can be quickly retrieved in a few seconds on the Internet. Mentors will be more successful by keeping these generational factors in mind, although the values and life goals of their mentees may differ.

Although mentoring is a valuable career development strategy for surgical residents, it should not be forced on a trainee. Residency Program Directors should conduct discussions with residents to educate them on the value of mentorship, and even be willing to help each resident identify mentors. However, the decision on entering a mentorship relationship should be the resident's personal choice without any form of coercion. Assigning a coach is different. The coach–coachee relationship is typically less close and more focused on a particular topic for which the trainee needs improvement. Requiring a surgical resident to accept coaching when needed is a sound approach to supporting a resident struggling in one area or another.

Learning to become a surgical specialist is a daunting journey and those responsible for providing the education and training toward helping an individual achieve that end carry a critically important responsibility. Surgeons serving society must be highly qualified and capable of performing with little room for error. Teachers of residents have the major responsibility for assuring the trainee learns the necessary knowledge and skills to become certified and hopefully boarded in their specialty. Role models and coaches can provide important guidance to budding surgeons; however, mentors can have the greatest impact on helping an otherwise average resident reach their full career and even life potential.

DISCLOSURE

The authors do not have any relationship with a commercial company that has a direct financial interest in the subject matter or materials discussed in the article or with a company making a competing product.

REFERENCES

1. Assael L. Every surgeon needs mentors: a Halstedian/Socratic model in the modern age. J Oral Maxillofac Surg 2010;68:1217–8.
2. Hupp JR. Two-way mentoring: learning from residents. J Oral Maxillofac Surg 2020;78:1–2.
3. The Origin of "Mentor" Comes Straight Out of Greek Mythology (And the Story's Epic. Available at: https://www.growthmentor.com/blog/origin-of-word-mentor/. Accessed January 20, 2022.
4. Healy NA, Cantillion P, Malone C, et al. Role models and mentors in surgery. Am J Surg 2012;204:256–61.
5. Halpern LR. The odyssey of mentoring: "from baby-boomer, to Millennial and beyond. Oral Maxillofacial Surg Clin N Am 2021;33(4):435–47.
6. Geraci SA, Thigpen SC. A review of mentoring in academic medicine. Am J Med Sci 2017;353(2):151–7.
7. Barondess JA. A brief history of mentoring. Trans Am Clin Climatol Assoc 1995;106:1–24.
8. Standing Committee for Postgraduate Medical and Dental Education. Supporting doctors and dentists at work: an inquiry into mentoring. London (UK): SCOPME; 1998.
9. Singletary SE. Mentoring surgeons for the 21st century. Ann Surg Oncol 2005;12:848–60.
10. Eby LT, Durley JR, Evans SC. Mentors' perceptions of negative mentoring experience: scale development and nomological validation. J Appl Psychol 2008;93:358–73.
11. Straus SE, Johnson MO, Marquez C, et al. Characteristics of successful and failed mentoring relationships: a qualitative study across two academic health centers. Acad Med 2013;88:82–9.
12. Atonoff MB, Varner ED, Yang SC, et al. Online learning in thoracic surgical training: promising results of a multi-institutional pilot study. Ann Thorac Surg 2014;98(3):1057–63.
13. Sambunjak D, Marusic A. Mentoring: what's in a name? J Am Med Assocc 2009;302(23):2591–2.
14. Rombeau J. What is mentoring and who is a mentor?. In: Rombeau J, Goldberg A, Loveland-Jones C, editors. Surgical mentoring: building tomorrow's leaders. New York: Springer Science + Business Media; 2010. p. 1–14.
15. Detsky AS, Baerlocher MD. Academic mentoring: how to give it and how to get it. J Am Med Assoc 2007;297(19):134–6.
16. Mulcahey MK, Waterman BR, Hart R, et al. The role of a mentoring in the development of successful orthopedic surgeons. J Am Acad Orthop Surg 2018; 26(123):463–71.
17. Zerzan JT, Hess R, Schur E, et al. Making the most of a mentor: a guide for mentees. Acad Med 2009; 84(1):140–4.
18. Welch J, Jimenez HL, Walthall J, et al. The woman in emergency mendicine mentoring program: an innovative approach to mentoring. J Grad Med Educat 2012;4(3):362–6.
19. Aggarwal A, Rosen CB, Nehemiah A, et al. Is there color or sex behind the mask and sterile blue? Examining sex and racial demographics within academic surgery. Ann Surg 2020;273:21–7.
20. Nellis JC, Eisele DW, Francis HW, et al. Impact of a mentored student clerkship on underrepresented minority diversity in otolaryngology-head and neck surgery. Laryngoscope 2016;126:2684–8.
21. Fagen M. The term mentor: a review of the literature and pragmatic solution. Into J Nurse 1988;2:508.
22. Bonrath EM, Dedy NJ, Gordon LE, et al. Comprehensive surgical coaching enhances surgical skill in the operating room: a randomized controlled trial. Ann Surg 2015;262(2):205–12.
23. Lin J, Reddy RM. Teaching, mentorship and coaching in surgical education. Thorac Surg Clin 2019;29: 311–20.
24. Asuka ES, Halari CA, Hakari MM. Mentoring in medicine: A retrospective review. ASRJETS 2016;19(1): 42–52.

The Role of Research Experiences in the Training of Oral and Maxillofacial Surgeons

Julie Glowacki, PhD

KEYWORDS

- Dental education • Research training • Oral & maxillofacial research • Critical thinking
- Professional education

KEY POINTS

- Critical thinking skills must be taught and reinforced at all levels of OMFS training and practice.
- Barriers to research experience during dental and postgraduate training include finding time and funding.
- Creative ways to expose trainees to active research and scholarship can improve critical thinking skills and help to retain clinician investigators in academic OMFS.

INTRODUCTION

There is growing attention and constant need to adapt curricula and faculty training in all health care disciplines because of substantial changes in the landscapes of clinical practices and health care delivery, expansion of biomedical and clinical knowledge, and introduction of innovative health care and educational technologies. These issues have been intensified by the global COVID-19 pandemic and escalating use of digital teaching tools. Responsibilities of the medical educator include the customary ones as a role model and source of knowledge and inspiration for trainees, but also concern new and changing methods of competency evaluation, principles of team management, professionalism, and maintaining a positive student-centered learning environment.[1] Many medical organizations stress the implementation of interprofessionalism in clinical practice and in education, which adds more requirements to the dental and oral surgery curricula.[2] In addition, there are deliberations about curriculum changes that would be needed to impart dental providers with expanded roles in basic, primary health care.[3–5]

There is a renewed emphasis on furthering life-long learning and critical thinking skills suitable for the often-erroneous web-based resources that overwhelm patients and clinicians alike. Advances in adult learning theory and research are making their way into clinical education as well. This is especially so on the appreciation of the different learning styles of millennials and other generations and of trainees' developmental stages.[6,7]

Critical thinking skills are vital for clinicians to make judgments, solve problems, and be creative when solutions are not obvious (**Fig. 1**). It is clear that critical thinking is essential for evidence-based practice and for establishing what rightly serves as guiding evidence.[8] Optimizing patient care algorithms is a life-time process that requires a rational and critical reassessment of the literature especially in light of experiences. Active critical thinking is needed to determine how to apply practice guidelines and also to help trainees recognize patients who are "outliers" and how to address their diagnoses and treatment.[9] A further benefit of critical thinking habits is for students to recognize and how to deal with ambiguity and uncertainty in clinical practice. It can also inspire

Department of Orthopedic Surgery, Brigham and Women's Hospital, Harvard Medical School, Harvard School of Dental Medicine, 75 Francis Street, Boston, MA 02115, USA
E-mail address: jglowacki@bwh.harvard.edu

Oral Maxillofacial Surg Clin N Am 34 (2022) 577–583
https://doi.org/10.1016/j.coms.2022.03.005
1042-3699/22/© 2022 Elsevier Inc. All rights reserved.

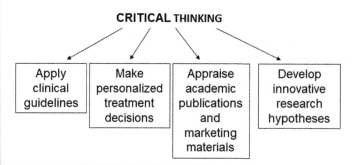

CRITICAL THINKING

Apply clinical guidelines

Make personalized treatment decisions

Appraise academic publications and marketing materials

Develop innovative research hypotheses

Fig. 1. Some responsibilities of clinicians that require highly developed critical thinking skills.

original hypotheses and creative research plans to address gaps in knowledge.

There is little in the literature about the role of research experiences in developing sharp critical thinking skills. The thesis of this article is that research experiences provide learners with powerful, discerning critical thinking skills that can serve a successful professional lifetime in private practice or in academia. Active participation in bench research, epidemiologic studies, and clinical trials have common benefits for clinicians at all career levels. Conducting literature reviews teach levels of evidence, how statistics can be used and misused, how to frame a hypothesis, how to design research plans to rigorously test the hypothesis, and how to excel in scientific writing. Ownership of a project or part of a project instills in early-stage trainees a sense of confidence, pride, and expertise from delving deeply into a subject area. Refining specific research skill-sets and understanding the limitations of methods and data interpretation further enhance the ability to judge publications and marketing materials.

RESEARCH EXPERIENCES FOR DENTAL STUDENTS

Accreditation bodies drive changes in curricula deemed important as health care systems evolve and innovative teaching methods develop. The policy statement made by the American Dental Education Association (ADEA) about dental research in the dental curriculum is explicit, namely to "(t)each the value, design, and methodology of dental research so that graduates may evaluate research findings and apply them to their practices."[10] Many groups throughout the world recognize the importance of research experiences as essential for dental education curricula to ensure that dentistry and its specialties remain scientifically, evidence-based professions.[11] Dental schools need to find creative solutions to the limitations that time and funding place on students' engagement in research projects.

There is information about research requirements for dental students at various institutions. Most of the studies on the value of research experiences in predoctoral dental students include detailed questionnaires to the trainees. A 2011 report from Istanbul describes the outcomes of the Student Scientific Research Club over a 15-year period.[12] The club was organized by student volunteers; no academic grades were given to participants, who elected to join the club and conduct research in their free time. Analysis showed higher Grade Point Averages on graduation for club members (n = 88) than for the rest of their classmates (n = 1267), but this could be explained by self-selection. Participating students believed that their classroom learning had evolved less by rote and more by reasoning and understanding, but those opinions were not compared with nonclub members. Club members viewed the research as important for their career development. They had a strong sense of independent inquiry skills and improved public speaking abilities as result of their research project. They valued developing relationships with faculty and a higher percentage of applicants for subsequent PhD programs were accepted for those applicants who were club members (52.6%) than were nonclub members (13.5%).

Five years of graduating classes from the Harvard School of Dental Medicine (HSDM) were surveyed anonymously for opinions about the then-recently adopted research requirement.[13] The study evaluated students who were in graduating classes from 2008 to 2012. Only 48% said they would definitely have pursued research even if it was not compulsory, but 83% said that they expect to have some involvement in research during their careers. A 7-month course was introduced to educate students about designing research protocols, proposal writing, research methodologies, statistical analyses, and presentations. An extension of the HSDM study covering the graduating classes of 2008 to 2017 reported a class-dependent variation between 58% and 87% of graduates judging the research component as positive and that 82%

expected to remain involved with research in some capacity.[14]

Institutions of various types have initiated different ways to enhance research training for dental students. Tufts University School of Dental Medicine created a selective Student Summer Research Program with stipends and the Dean's Research Honors Scholarship with 5 tuition scholarships.[15] Those programs addressed the obstacles of protected time and student debt to some degree, and they promoted a culture of student research likely to affect academic career decisions of involved graduates. The Marquette University School of Dentistry launched a curriculum that supported student research and scholarly activity throughout all 4 years with a new curriculum.[16] It integrated research into the curriculum and may serve as a model for research-nonintensive institutions intending to increase student interest in academic and research careers. The program included research mentors from all parts of Marquette University for 1- to 3-month periods of research and for more intensive options. The program was possible because of two federal grants for faculty salaries, faculty development, technology, and curriculum materials.

A nationwide online survey was distributed to US dental students in 2012.[17] A striking finding was that 63% had conducted research before matriculation at a US dental school. This supports undergraduates' impression that having a research background may enhance success in applying to dental school. Respondents with research experiences as dental students had greater appreciation of the role of research in evidence-based practices and of the importance of research in dental education. Those dental students believed that there may be inadequate training in biostatistics and research methodologies.

The exact role of research in the education of dental students remains under discussion because of the obstacles of time and funding. Bertolami emphasized the great importance of developing intellectual rigor and scholarship in students because it is necessary that they "will be able to acquire and assimilate new knowledge and to adapt to the changes in practice and in the profession that the future requires."[18]

There continues to be a need for well-qualified faculty to attain the educational, clinical, and research missions of dental schools. A survey of US oral sciences PhD program graduates showed that 35% of such graduates became faculty in US academic institutions and 13% became faculty in non-US institutions.[19] Unfortunately, the analysis showed that only 3.9% of vacant US faculty

positions were filled by those graduates, and a minority were DDS/PhD holders. A more recent analysis of these programs was not retrievable; nevertheless, the suggestion is that other solutions to the loss of academic talent need to be sought.

RESEARCH EXPERIENCES FOR ORAL AND MAXILLOFACIAL SURGERY RESIDENTS

Knowledge about biostatistics arose in a study of OMFS residents' understanding of data analysis and interpretation of research results.[20] A questionnaire that had been used for internal medicine residents was modified with OMFS examples. More than 90% of the responding OMFS residents reported having taken a biostatistics or epidemiology course and claimed to know the subject matter. Despite that confidence, they scored very poorly (38%) in basic questions about variables, statistical significance, and types of research studies. Reinforcement of that learning during residency and thereafter seems to be needed.

A 2011 report of questionnaires sent to 101 US program directors and all residents about research during OMFS training indicated that only 36% of programs provided scheduled research time, most often 3 months or less.[21] Most program directors and residents responded that research projects may be of value for those considering an academic career, but not for those entering private practice. They commented that short research experiences are likely not sufficient for residents with academic aspirations to develop the mindset necessary for them to advance in the OMFS field in future years. Those beliefs do not seem to recognize the importance of a solid foundation in, and regular refreshing of critical thinking skills throughout any clinical career (see **Fig. 1**). If properly designed, research experiences can enhance critical thinking skills and habits of questioning dogmas in the most fulfilling surgical careers.

There is little doubt that adult learning principles, self-directed life-learning skills, and ability to adapt to changes, such as those presented in the information age, should be reinforced during the training of OMFS residents.[22] Opinions are divided about research requirements for OMFS residents entering private practice.[21] Activities other than research activities that provide scholarly activity and intellectual growth are already components of resident training, for example, teaching conferences, quality care conferences, grand rounds, interdisciplinary conferences, and journal clubs.[23] Some specific recommendations for journal clubs are offered later in discussion.

There is information from other surgical specialties germane to the professional value of research experiences during training. A survey of 1495 academic otolaryngologists revealed that those with formal research training had greater publication h-indices, more NIH funding, and higher academic rank.[24] Those outcomes were significantly greater for those with a PhD degree or completion of a research fellowship. Those metrics of academic success are likely to be related to having greater impact on advancing the field. A similar, small study of 299 full-time academic OMF surgeons showed increased NIH funding by those with formal research training or advanced degrees (PhD, DMSc, DPH, DPhil, ScD).[25] They also had greater publication h-indices, but there was no difference in current academic rank. A cross-sectional study of 927 current academic plastic surgeons with subspecialty fellowship training (35.6% hand, 32.0% craniofacial, and 28.1% microsurgery) found a significant impact on research productivity, academic rank, and leadership (residency director or chair).[26] A large survey of academic plastic surgeons showed that 34.4% of those serving leadership roles in national plastic surgery societies held dual degrees, as did 29.2% in leadership roles in local/regional societies; those percents contrasted with an overall 16% without dual degrees.[27] It is noted that the MBA degree had the greatest association with leadership.

The recent decade-long rise in the number of applicants to integrated plastic surgery programs was reported to be associated with increased emphasis of applicants on research productivity and a dedicated year of research, typically after the third year of medical school.[28] Data showed a 97% match for those with a research year, compared with 81% without the year. Applicants' publication records contributed to the difference. Another group concluded that those applicants without access to a coveted, funded research opportunity, especially in the face of medical school debt, are thus at a disadvantage.[29] The authors speculated that information about such research opportunities is less available to minority applicants in research-nonintensive schools and that this pipeline matter needs attention. Another pipeline problem has been identified in academic plastic surgery, with a low percent of leadership roles with women despite a growing percent in faculty positions and as members in professional societies.[30]

PERSPECTIVE AND RECOMMENDATIONS

In addition to this commentary on literature about research requirements in dental and OMFS training programs as well as those in diverse surgical training programs, the author's personal experience and observations from an academic biomedical research career can offer realistic perspectives on this topic. A brief description of her research training philosophy and programs provides not only an outlook sharpened over decades but also offers scrutinized and tested recommendations for consideration.

Clinical advances in dentistry and in OMFS, as in all specialties, follow from progress in clinical or basic research that targets a specific problem in a rigorous, hypothesis-driven manner. Typically, a clinician would pose a clinical question that is encountered during the care of patients. This person is often described as a "clinical champion" because of the massive commitment that is necessary to carry the research forward with essential collaborators and funding. When the inquisitive clinician champion is a faculty member, other institutional colleagues can be recruited to form a team that assesses the feasibility and develops a research plan to test the hypothesis. If needed methods are outside the experience of the budding team, collaborators at other institutions may be sought. Members of the team can be dispatched to laboratories that will train them in specific research methodology. The clinical champion in private practice may contribute to the enterprise by asking thoughtful, insightful questions at a seminar or convention that spurs an academic team to pursue the matter.

Grand Rounds and conference presentations that are explicitly designed to convey the impact of innovative research on clinical dogmas and transformations in clinical care can show residents how each of them could make a difference. Inspiring narratives and an open culture of asking questions can reinforce critical ruminating as a life-long habit. PhD researchers' participation in discussions at those activities can extend the learning to potentially new research ideas.

A valuable way to make advances in solving OMFS problems is to build collaborations between full-time research scientists and clinical investigators. Busy clinicians can rarely find the time to supervise laboratory personnel and write grant applications. PhDs with a desire to contribute to biomedical research can find a rewarding career by teaming with an inquisitive clinician investigator. Both need to be generous and respectful of the other. The PhD needs to be patient in explaining the strengths and weaknesses of research methodologies. The clinical champion needs to be patient and respectful in explaining the clinical problem and failed attempts to solve them. Recruitment of a creative PhD scientist requires explicit discussions about authorship and academic promotions as well as the responsibilities expected to earn those career rewards, such as background literature review of the topic, formulating multiple testable hypotheses, feasibility testing of new methods, writing grant applications, supervising students and technicians in the laboratory, and assuring the rigor and quality of data and interpretations.

There are several recognizable difficulties to make a productive team of a basic scientist with a clinical champion. One is that recent PhD graduates often feel far too secure in continuing research on their thesis topic and using only familiar research tools and methodologies. Moving into an unfamiliar research topic requires a great deal of background study and mastery of unfamiliar topics. They may not have the intellectual flexibility and fundamental training to join a biomedical research team. A prevailing banality is that surgeons consider PhD researchers to be used as assisting technicians; on the other hand, it is commonly presumed that PhD researchers deem surgeons as inferior thinkers with good eye–hand coordination. Indeed, there are PhD researchers who are content to be technicians and carry out experiments in exchange for secure, nonacademic positions. Clear expectations of each other's contributions and mutual respect are required for success. Another hurdle to overcome is terminology. The PhD collaborator can benefit enormously from regular attendance at Grand Rounds. Such exposure expands the understanding of diagnostic criteria, surgical planning, outcome measures, and the state of evidence-based practice for the range OMFS problems. It is disheartening to hear from departmental leadership in all surgical specialties that it can be difficult to require that PhD scientists attend Grand Rounds which often are scheduled in the early morning or early evening hours. Recording lectures for later viewing is an easy solution to that limitation.

Surgical specialties are especially amenable to research with animal models. Surgical trainees enjoy learning to operate on research animals. Despite the limitations of applying findings from animal models to clinical recommendations, carefully designed surgical models can be valuable for testing bone graft substitutes for example. In the early stages of research with limited funding, rodent models can be designed and validated for answering specific questions about tissue responses to implant materials.[31–36] More costly research animals, such as the Yucatan minipig require greater levels of funding. The minipig is good for OMFS research for an array of anatomic and biological features.[37,38] Its bone turnover rate in the mandible is equal to that of humans, whereas other research species have more rapid turnover and heal bone defects too rapidly. The pig temporo-mandibular joint is similar to that of the human in that its motion has both rotational and translational components. In addition, the chewing pattern and transmission of chewing forces to the midface through the zygomatic buttresses and piriform apertures are similar in minipigs and humans. A series of publications on distraction osteogenesis in the minipig mandible[37–40] and maxilla[41] provided preclinical research and validation of new devices subsequently used in patients.

The publications about distraction osteogenesis in the minipig[37–40,42] make additional points about OMFS research. The lists of authors indicate the array of specialists that can be needed for different components of the program's research. Several articles also represent small, ancillary studies that can be assigned to trainees.[39,40] Another way to engage trainees for short-term research assignments can be to have them learn new methodology, for example, gene expression analysis by reverse transcriptase-polymerase chain reaction assays, while repeating work of others for reproducibility; doing so allows the team to indicate in publications that the studies were repeated 2 or 3 times. Such short-term laboratory work can generate a trainee's abstract and presentation of the work. With experience, the PhD researcher can compile a list of achievable assignments for summer students. Along with a customized reading list and data review sessions, such short-term assignments can prove successful to stimulate a novice to further research.

An original line of research was initiated when an OMFS clinical champion and PhD colleague shared training a summer dental student. They realized that the surgeon had access to excess, discarded pediatric marrow available for research along the line of research the PhD was conducting with adult cells. After obtaining consent to anonymize and study the cells, they discovered that the pediatric cells had the capacity to activate vitamin D and thereby have their differentiation to osteoblasts be stimulated by vitamin D precursors[43,44]. These are the only retrievable reports of research with pediatric marrow-derived stem cells, likely because of the unique research team.

Another important role of the PhD collaborator is to train OMFS residents in the latest knowledge relevant to surgery; this may entail frequent didactic updates in bone biology and pathophysiology, in effects of aging and systemic disease on surgical outcomes, and in ongoing research in the department's laboratory. It is advisable that the

PhD presenter learn to insert suitable clinical "pearls" every 3 to 5 minutes during such a lecture to help a clinical audience connect new knowledge to existing knowledge. Other Socratic tools, like asking the audience probing and leading questions, can assure active learning.

Judicious management of journal clubs ought to include frequent discussion of weak and poorly designed publications. Of course, a journal club ought to be used to expose residents to the latest, best publications that have a great impact on patient care. Some journal clubs discuss only top articles from top journals. This is not optimal for learning about poor evidence. Discussion of publications with inappropriate statistical methods, for example, teaches the residents that bad articles can be published, and how they can learn to gauge the quality of evidence and justification of conclusions. Half of the meeting time should be devoted to discussing the weaknesses in a publication and what next steps of research are indicated. These skills apply to marketing materials, which can also be discussed in journal clubs. A professor's invitation to residents to co-review articles, with the permission of the journal and the understanding of confidentiality, is especially powerful to hone trainees' critical reading competency.

SUMMARY

Changes in health care delivery and technology require adjustments to dental and residency training. Critical thinking and life-long learning skills must be taught and reinforced at all levels of OMFS training and practice because they are essential for best clinical practices. Research experiences provide active learning about critical thought processes in different contexts and refine learners' abilities to judge publications and marketing materials. Barriers to research experiences during dental and postgraduate training include time and funding. Surveys indicate that dental graduates expect to have some involvement in research during their careers, but those aspirations are often not achieved even for some in academics. Strong partnerships between PhD researchers and OMFS clinical investigators, formed to advance the field, can also have an impact on trainees' involvement in research and their understanding of rigorous evidence-based principles of clinical care. Creative ways to expose trainees to active research and scholarship can improve critical thinking skills and help to recruit and retain clinician investigators in academic OMFS.

DISCLOSURE

The authors have nothing to disclose.

REFERENCES

1. Schindler BA. The clinician as educator: Redefining the medical educator's role and toolbox. In: Gotian R, Kang Y, Safdieh J, editors. Handbook of research on the efficacy of training programs and systems in medical education. Hershey (PA): IGI Global, Medical Information Science Reference; 2020. p. 345–55.
2. Kaste LM, Halpern LR. The alphabet soup of interprofessional education and collaborative practice acronyms with dental seasoning. Dent Clin North Am 2016;60:xiii–xvi.
3. Donoff RB, Daley GQ. Oral health care in the 21st century: It is time for the integration of dental and medical education. J Dent Educ 2020;84:999–1002.
4. Lamster IB, Myers-Wright N. Oral health care in the future: expansion of the scope of dental practice to improve health. J Dent Educ 2017;81:eS83–90.
5. Kaste LM, Wilder JR, Halpern LR, et al. Emerging topics for dentists as primary care providers. Dent Clin North Am 2013;57(2):371–6. Available at: https://doi.org/10.3389/fdmed.2021.703958. Accessed January 30, 2022.
6. Lam HT, O'Toole TG, Arola PE, et al. Factors associated with the satisfaction of millennial generation dental residents. J Dent Educ 2012;76:1416–26.
7. Velez DR. Modern didactic formats in surgery: a systematic review. Am Surg 2022. 31348221074252.
8. Mercuri M, Baigrie BS. What counts as evidence in an evidence-based world? J Eval Clin Pract 2019;25:533–5.
9. Mercuri M, Sherbino J, Sedran RJ, et al. When guidelines don't guide: the effect of patient context on management decisions based on clinical practice guidelines. Acad Med 2015;90:191–6.
10. ADEA Policy Statements: Recommendations and guidelines for academic dental institutions. Available at: https://www.adea.org/about_adea/governance. Accessed January 30, 2022.
11. Emrick JJ, Gullard A. Integrating research into dental student training: a global necessity. J Dent Res 2013;92:1053–5.
12. Guven Y, Uysal O. The importance of student research projects in dental education. Eur J Dent Educ 2011;15:90–7.
13. Nalliah RP, Lee MK, Da Silva JD, et al. Impact of a research requirement in a dental school curriculum. J Dent Educ 2014;78:1364–71.
14. Van der Groen TA, Olsen BR, Park SE. Effects of a research requirement for dental students: a

retrospective analysis of students' perspectives across ten years. J Dent Educ 2018;82:1171–7.

15. Doherty EH, Karimbux NY, Kugel G. Creation and initial outcomes of a selective four-year research program for predoctoral dental students. J Dent Educ 2016;80:1405–12.

16. Iacopino AM, Lynch DP, Taft T. Preserving the pipeline: a model dental curriculum for research non-intensive institutions. J Dent Educ 2004;68:44–9.

17. Holman SD, Wietecha MS, Gullard A, et al. U.S. dental students' attitudes toward research and science: impact of research experience. J Dent Educ 2014;78:334–48.

18. Bertolami CN. The role and importance of research and scholarship in dental education and practice. J Dent Educ 2002;66:918–24.

19. Herzog CR, Berzins DW, DenBesten P, et al. Oral sciences PhD program enrollment, graduates, and placement: 1994 to 2016. J Dent Res 2018;97:483–91.

20. Best AM, Laskin DM. Oral and maxillofacial surgery have poor understanding of biostatistics. J Oral Maxillofac Surg 2013;71:227–34.

21. Mohammad AE, Best AM, Laskin DM. Attitudes and opinions of residency directors and residents about the importance of research in oral and maxillofacial surgery residencies. J Oral Maxillofac Surg 2011;69:2064–9.

22. Carlson ER. Lifelong learning and professional development. J Oral Maxillofac Surg 2016;74:875–6.

23. Hupp JR. Research during residency - should it be mandated? J Oral Maxillofac Surg 2011;69:2685–7.

24. Bobian MR, Shah N, Svider PF, et al. Laryngoscope 2017;127:E15–21.

25. Han JT, Egbert MA, Dodson TB, et al. Is formal research training associated with academic success in Oral and Maxillofacial Surgery? J Oral Maxillofac Surg 2018;76:27–33.

26. Egro FM, Smith BT, Murphy CP, et al. The impact of fellowship training in academic plastic surgery. Ann Plast Surg 2021;87:461–6.

27. Pyfer BJ, Hernandez JA, Glener AD, et al. leadership and advanced degrees: Evaluating the association between dual degrees and leadership roles in academic plastic surgery. Ann Plast Surg 2022;88:118–21.

28. Mellia JA, Mauch JT, Broach RB, et al. Moving the goalposts: Inequity concerns regarding research years and the integrated plastic surgery match. Plast Reconstr Surg 2021;148:1086e–7.

29. Zimmerman CE, Humphries LS, Taylor JA. Equitable access to research opportunities in plastic surgery: development of a research fellowship database. Plast Reconstr Surg 2021;148:1087e–8.

30. Chen W, Baron M, Bourne DA, et al. A report on the representation of women in academic plastic surgery leadership. Plast Reconstr Surg 2020;145:844–52.

31. Kaban LB, Glowacki J, Murray JE. Repair of experimental mandibular bony defects in rats. Surg Forum 1979;30:519–21.

32. Kaban LB, Glowacki J. Induced osteogenesis in the repair of experimental mandibular defects in rats. J Dent Res 1981;60:1356–64.

33. Mulliken JB, Kaban LB, Glowacki J. Induced osteogenesis–the biological principle and clinical applications. J Surg Res 1984;37:487–96.

34. Kaban LB, Glowacki J. Augmentation of rat mandibular ridge with demineralized bone implants. J Dent Res 1984;63:998–1002.

35. Pettis GY, Kaban LB, Glowacki J. Tissue response to composite ceramic hydroxyapatite/demineralized bone implants. J Oral Maxillofac Surg 1990;48:1068–74.

36. Glowacki J, Schulten AJ, Perrott D, et al. Nicotine impairs distraction osteogenesis in the rat mandible. Int J Oral Maxillofac Surg 2008;37:156–61.

37. Troulis MJ, Glowacki J, Perrott DH, et al. Effects of latency and rate on bone formation in a porcine mandibular distraction model. J Oral Maxillofac Surg 2000;58:507–13.

38. Glowacki J, Shusterman EM, Troulis M, et al. Distraction osteogenesis of the porcine mandible: histomorphometric evaluation of bone. Plast Reconstr Surg 2004;113:566–73.

39. Yates KE, Troulis MJ, Kaban LB, et al. IGF-I, TGF-beta, and BMP-4 are expressed during distraction osteogenesis of the pig mandible. Int J Oral Maxillofac Surg 2002;31:173–8.

40. Castaño FJ, Troulis MJ, Glowacki J, et al. Proliferation of masseter myocytes after distraction osteogenesis of the porcine mandible. J Oral Maxillofac Surg 2001;59:302–7.

41. Papadaki ME, Troulis MJ, Glowacki J, et al. A minipig model of maxillary distraction osteogenesis. J Oral Maxillofac Surg 2010;68:2783–91.

42. Kaban LB, Seldin EB, Kikinis R, et al. Clinical application of curvilinear distraction osteogenesis for correction of mandibular deformities. J Oral Maxillofac Surg 2009;67:996–1008.

43. Ruggiero B, Padwa BL, Christoph KM, et al. Vitamin D metabolism and regulation in pediatric MSCs. J Steroid Biochem Mol Biol. 2016;164:287–91.

44. Li J, Padwa BL, Zhou S, et al. Synergistic effect of $1\alpha,25$-dihydroxyvitamin D_3 and 17β-estradiol on osteoblast differentiaion of pediatric MSCs. J Steroid Biochem Mol Biol 2018;177:103–8.

Artificial Intelligence in Oral and Maxillofacial Surgery Education

Deepak G. Krishnan, DDS

KEYWORDS

- Artificial intelligence in medicine (AIM) • Machine learning • Deep learning • Future of education

KEY POINTS

- Artificial intelligence (AI) is a branch of computer science that is focused on creating programs, algorithms, and machines that can potentially think and function independently.
- Medical education follows trends in medical practice adopting AI.
- Oral and maxillofacial surgical practice and education are a natural niche for AI to insert its adaptability.
- AI will improve the diagnosis of disease, training of surgeons, and improve patient outcomes based on its ability to predict patterns.

INTRODUCTION

Artificial intelligence (AI) is a broad academic branch of computer science focused on creating systems that are capable of intelligent and independent function. The concept of machines having the capacity to think and act like humans has been in existence beyond science fiction since the 1950s, with ebbs and flow in the momentum of development of the actual science.

For a computer program to replicate human behavior and interactions, machines and programs that are capable of speech recognition, natural language and image processing, robotics, and pattern recognition are being developed. When that program is given a "body" it is referred to as a haptic unit or a robot. Machines can be programmed to be impeccably skillful at pattern recognition. Algorithms and programs have been developed that allow the system to analyze data, identify patterns in data and even make decisions with minimal human intervention. This is called Machine Learning—a subset of AI. The basic premise of machine learning is to replicate the structure and function of the human brain and its neural network, with the intent of replicating its cognitive capabilities in

machines. It seems like a natural extension of current technology whereby smaller chips have the capability of processing larger databases of information. When a series of algorithms are all looking for patterns within the same data set (imagine a massive data set), they can be useful in predicting models of outcomes, reliably. An interconnected network resembles synapses in the human brain and is referred to as a neural network.

Deep learning in machines is currently possible making machines savvy to process patterns, see and hear, and have some memory of the immediate past events. In theory, machines can process much more data than human process and maintain them in their neural network. Machines can process this data and predict patterns of behavior based on what it has learned. Machines can learn from errors and will never repeat that error. Machines can decipher complex patterns and learn more than humans are ever capable of learning. They can look at lots of high-dimensional data and determine patterns. The factor of subjective human error is eliminated with the machines performing the same task. Once it learns these patterns, it can make predictions that humans cannot even come close to.

University of Cincinnati, Cincinnati Children's Hospital and Medical Center, 200 Albert Sabin Way, Cincinnati, OH 45242, USA
E-mail address: deepak.krishnan@uc.edu

Oral Maxillofacial Surg Clin N Am 34 (2022) 585–591
https://doi.org/10.1016/j.coms.2022.03.006
1042-3699/22/© 2022 Elsevier Inc. All rights reserved.

AI is becoming ubiquitous in daily life. At the time of writing this article, global wireless connectivity is at its fifth generation -5G-iteration. This allows for data to be transmitted over wireless broadband Internet connections at peak speeds of up to 20 gigabits per second. The gigabit is a multiple of the unit bit for digital information storage. 1 gigabit $= 10^9$ bits $= 1000000000$ bits. This allows for seamless and fast interconnectivity of different devices via the Internet allowing them to send and receive data from each other—a concept called the Internet of Things (IoT). This is the ability of your mattress with sensors to alert your wearable device about the quality of your sleep and your coffee maker to alert your refrigerator that you are running low on milk and for your refrigerator to alert your car to remind you to pick up milk from the grocer on your next trip. It is estimated that by 2025, 100 million devices will connect to each other and currently perhaps there are about 6 to 15 devices in most US households seeking your attention unless you physically turn them off.[1]

The fact that your mobile phone has the intelligence to ask you if you would like "all notifications turned off for the next 1 hour" because it senses that your calendar has a meeting on the schedule for that hour is the result of AI taking over to silence the interruptions of technology. This is the ability of the system to have context awareness like a human mind. At some point in the (near) future, AI will silence all technology and suppress them to whereby it will no longer be friction but will add value to your life and make it simpler. Interestingly, this kind of AI or digital revolution will make current or future technology transparent in our lives by immersing us in it even more.

AI will grow into every aspect of human existence including creativity and philosophy and most certainly education. Modern medical and surgical educators will embrace AI without even realizing that they are doing so consciously. Technology has already altered our daily practice of medicine in the last couple of decades exponentially. It is only natural that the student of the day also adapts to this sea change and learns contemporaneously. AI is not a futuristic concept anymore but an unavoidable article in medical education now.

ARTIFICIAL INTELLIGENCE IN EDUCATION

The Coronavirus pandemic (2020–2022) forced several sectors of our civilization to evolve and adapt. Education quickly pivoted to online forums globally with virtual platforms and mobile phones transforming into classrooms. It revolutionized both teaching and learning. Experts are predicting that the use of AI in the education sector will grow by 47.77% by 2025.[2] Nearly all aspects of AI—machine learning, natural language processing, and deep learning will all help solve learning challenges in all sectors of education whether K-12 or higher education or consumer education. AI is expected to help customize learning, especially in emerging markets whereby learning disabilities and languages are challenges. There will be an emphasis on chatbots and new markets that have previously been off-limits for traditional education. Global AI usage in education is expected to reach $5.8 billion in investment by 2025.[2]

As in many other industries, the utility of AI in task automation will become handy in education as well. The need for a human to fulfill administrative and organizational tasks in a classroom can essentially be eliminated by using AI. Most of the nonteaching tasks that are often considered overwhelming and distracting by teachers can easily be assigned to technology. An argument can be made that objective grading, task assignments, and evaluations including complex psychometrics can be conducted better by a computer program rather than a tired teacher. No more teacher's pets!

Adaptive learning is a strong suit for AI already. Software designed for games, and programs already exist. AI is particularly adept at identifying the preferences and interests of its users. An example of personalized prioritization is how websites of companies such as Amazon and Netflix function—offering you other products, movies, or shows for your consideration based on your current choices. This personalization can be applied to education. AI can make learning more comfortable and smoother for especially those that have learning disabilities through custom-tailoring. It will understand patterns of each student's learning capacity, challenges and weaknesses, and strengths arguably better than a human teacher. It will be able to tailor learning modules based on the student's ability, agility, and availability. Teachers will be a support system, ensuring that the AI is functional and will be available to students when they need a personal instruction. The near future, at least, suggests a hybrid classroom.

AI will also make education globally accessible and invalidate the challenges of different languages including visual impairment. Already, email platforms and presentation software such as PowerPoint can navigate easily between languages and AI further strengthens real-time translations and transcripts. This includes the ability of using AI-powered chatbots or software applications used in "virtual assistant" conversations that replicates a human's response either in an on-line chat or a text-to-speech making available a 24/7 teacher for the student. This again eliminates challenges in global classrooms with time zones and languages.

AI will likely bridge the gap between content taught and applications in real life in many fields. Abstract ideas and impractical curricula can be analyzed in real-world application scenarios creating smart content modules making both teaching and learning realistic and practical. This will especially be true in medical education as will be discussed later. The learners themselves are becoming savvy in their studying. AI can help generate bite-sized learning, web-based curricula, digital study guides, and project management making studying easier. Assignment writing ser-vices, web-based study environments, and simu-lation of skills, visualization of concepts using augmented reality (AR) and virtual reality (VR) are already available to the modern student. Content can easily be kept track of and updated regularly without human involvement.

Pattern recognition will allow teachers and the class to look at strengths and weaknesses of groups, subgroups, and individuals in each cohort or classroom. AI will have the ability to identify the part of the study material that is perceived as tough or easy, questions that are psychometrically valid or invalid, and predict trends in student per-formance as well as curriculum/teacher effective-ness without subjective bias. Essentially AI will not eliminate teachers but complement them and hold them accountable for performing at the best teaching practices.

ARTIFICIAL INTELLIGENCE IN MEDICAL EDUCATION

In a 2019 study that sought to understand medi-cal students' attitude and understanding of AI, especially in Radiology, 71% agreed on the need for AI to be included in medical training and 83% disagreed with statements that human radiologists will be replaced by an AI bot.[3] Studies have shown similar results in Canadian students,[4] and Ireland.[5] The potential for inte-grating AI in medicine (AIM) is being realized at an unprecedented pace with regulatory bodies such as the FDA creating action plan documents on the topic—"Artificial Intelligence/Machine Learning (AI/ML)-Based Software as a Medical Device (SaMD) Action Plan."[6] FDA acknowledges that "artificial intelligence and machine learning technologies have the potential to transform health care by deriving new and important in-sights from the vast amount of data generated

during the delivery of health care every day" and has created 10 guiding principles for the same and is welcoming constant feedback from all stake-holders at https://www.regulations.gov/docket/FDA-2019-N-1185 indefinitely.[7]

With industry and AIM moving ahead, discus-sions on the integration of medical informatics, AIM, and medical education are prevalent both at institutional as well as global scale.[8] As mentioned earlier, the pandemic forced all educa-tion to adapt to virtual and remote learning prac-tices and medical education was also an early adopter of this trend. Internet-based e-learning has its limitations and it became quickly evident in clinical behavior and patient outcomes exposing some of the nuances of teaching patient–physician interactions.[9] To formalize the integration of AI into the pedagogical method of medical education, attempts have begun as was discussed in detail by Owolabi in his recent article.[10] They have proposed "a framework that can help to optimize the introduction and use of innovations and educational technology in the de-livery of medical education."

Most medical schools are looking at integrating mixed reality technologies (augmented, virtual and hybrid) into the teaching of anatomy, radiology, surgery, pathology, and physiology among others. Industry has quickly caught up to the demand. Vir-tual cadavers and integration of 3D imaging into anatomic specimens have come way beyond their prototypical models. Gamification of concepts of pathophysiology allows for the visualization of ab-stract concepts in biochemistry for instance, mak-ing both teaching and learning of these concepts easier. While in theory that seems like a good idea, in actuality, a recent study shows that there are few plans or implementations reported on how to incorporate AI into the medical curriculum in the US.[11]

As an application of AI in clinical medicine be-comes more commonplace, medical students are getting exposed to AI on the job even if training is not formal. Robotic surgery, digital surgical plan-ning, medical applications and software, intuitive electronic health record systems, and other tech-nological immersion expose them plenty to the concepts of how technologies such as AI influence patient care. AI can easily be incorporated into in-terpretations of studies like ECG, Echo, labora-tories, among others, and play a major role in predicting probabilities in the care of the patient and treatment outcomes.[12] Robotic surgery has become commonplace in many surgical subspe-cialties. The next generation of robots is expected to incorporate machine learning correcting user errors and making positioning decisions and incorporating digital planning. Surgical management algorithms and decision processes (eg, the Markov decision process of keloid management) are low-hanging fruit for the development of AI algorithms and treatment models.

However, regardless of such noteworthy potential, we seem to not have completely embraced AI into our daily practice. Despite an AI revolution in most fields including health care, public health, and education, medical education currently seems to have some realistic challenges in taking advantage of the offerings of AI. Clinicians who take on the role of academicians often lack formal education in teaching. Even the preclinical educators in medical and dental schools lack the expertise to teach AI in the context of medicine. The potential for using machine learning and deep learning as a quantitative assessment tool is overlooked. In theory, skills training, especially in surgeons can be evaluated by reviewing videos of a procedure focusing on the quality of steps as performed by a novice relative to a skilled master surgeon may allow the identification of areas for intervention/improvement.[13]

Admittedly, we are at the very nascent stages of adoption of this technology, and it might take several iterations of collaborations between physician educators, educators, and content experts in AI, to incorporate AI into medical education to its fullest potential. The fear of physician and physician educator replacement by machines may be a barrier to the adoption of this technology. There is an inherent skepticism toward emerging technology, especially machine autonomy and a lack of trust. Then there is the resistance to curriculum change in institutions and regulatory bodies. The marketplace and nonmedical industry are bound to drive the change and medical education is likely to adapt through the influence of external forces when students show up to clinics with digital stethoscopes and apps that track patient trends and outcomes. Implementation of AIM will likely drive the change in medical education. The empowered patient seeking quicker and more advanced solutions may question the traditional approach to disease diagnosis and management. New diseases of the techno-world such as virtual posttraumatic stress disorder (v-PTSD)—a diagnosis for gamers who participate in virtual wars wearing VR goggles who experience similar symptoms as those soldiers who fought in real wars, or videogame epilepsy, or "text-neck" (neck pain from looking down at your phone, or wireless devices too frequently and for too long) will need new approaches to management that our students must learn.

ARTIFICIAL INTELLIGENCE IN ORAL AND MAXILLOFACIAL SURGERY

Oral and maxillofacial surgery (OMS) has not been too far behind in climbing on to the bandwagon of AI.[14–16] As expected, the specialty has gravitated toward contemplations and predictions of potential applications in science-fictional robotics and use of machine learning in diagnosis and prognostication. A promising work of using neural networks in the diagnosis of temporomandibular joint internal derangement is an actual application of AI in OMS.[17] Machine learning has also been explored in the field of diagnosis of orofacial pain with some potential for future development.[18] Similar machine learning models have been reported to show "promising performances for diagnostic and prognostic analyses in studies of oral cancer"; again, some work in its infancy awaiting regulatory adoption.[19]

The concept of using AI to create prediction models is being developed globally to learn outcomes of diseases such as oral cavity tumors, patient survival and predict occult nodal metastasis.[19–21] Similar predictive models have been developed in poly-system trauma whereby machine learning helps create prognostic and outcomes calculators that can be extrapolated to facial injuries. Much of the manual work can be replaced in applications that require extensive assessments and landmark plotting such as in the functional assessment of facial nerve dysfunction.[22] These are steps toward automating a labor-intensive database and facial landmark localization models. Validated AI algorithms will take less time and are predictably more accurate than human plotting and assessments. Applications in the diagnosis of normal appearances and deviations from those normal seem like low-hanging fruit for the application of AI in OMS. Morphometric variations are easier and more predictably analyzed by AI than humans.[23]

The use of 3D printing and digital planning technology as well as robotics is already prevalent in OMS. This is just the tip of the iceberg as AI will start being incorporated into these existing technologic realms. Soon, machine learning will isolate patterns and preferences of individual surgeons, design of osteotomies, and personalize surgical plans without a 3rd party. 3D scanning technology will become more realistic and diagnostic and incorporate virtual or augmented realities. Patient education tools such as predictive models of postoperative appearance will become more realistic. Personalized recipes for enhanced recovery after surgery (ERAS) protocols will become the norm.

Third-party payers will not be too far behind. Objective data on individual providers, referral patterns, use of resources and so forth, will be mapped using machine learning and will become the new benchmarks for reimbursement. Medicolegal world will adapt to looking at new evidence using deep learning, exposing patterns of erratic or ideal behavior, minimizing subjective errors in reviews, and employing accurate standards of care while deliberating cases. The implications are endless.

AI IN ORAL AND MAXILLOFACIAL SURGERY EDUCATION

AI has not permeated the field of dental education as it has medical education, and nor has it entered routine dental practice. This may be due to (1) limited data availability, accessibility, structure, and comprehensiveness, (2) lacking methodological rigor and standards in their development, (3) and practical questions around the value and usefulness of these solutions, but also ethics and responsibility.[24] As one investigates the prospect of the introduction of AI into dental education, the modus operandum must be like that in medical education—introduce AI into clinical practice and then adapt your teaching the student about that application. That along with the incorporation of digital literacy will ensure that the future dental student is contemporary. Some of the same challenges in achieving this goal regarding subject matter expertise and trust discussed with medical education are probably accentuated in the world of dental education.

Unlike medicine, dentistry adopted simulation very early on. Simulated preclinical exercises in cavity and crown preparations and teeth setting ensured that the student is somewhat adept in clinical skills before being presented to the live patient. Advanced surgical training in OMS also relies on simulation routinely. Surgical trainees learn suturing, knot tying, and surgical approaches through simulation whether it is on a cadaver or a sim-lab. Saw-bone skulls allow for teaching of principles of fracture fixation and animal models help train micro-vascular anastomosis. In the United States, an extension of that simulation training is the incorporation of simulation into office anesthesia team training. This involves training the OMS and their office-based team(s) using a high-fidelity mannequin programmed for airway embarrassment and rescue. The American Association of Oral and Maxillofacial Surgeons (AAOMS) has mandated this type of simulation training to all its members to maintain skills and train as a team to strengthen the safety of patient care in their care-delivery model. Efforts are underway to incorporate machine learning into this process to allow individuals, groups, teams, states, and the association to look at this data meaningfully and to personalize training based on trends that may be seen. AI can be the natural next step in simulation technology.

AI has other applications in surgical education. Carla Pugh's work at Stanford University suggests using AI in evaluating intraoperative events in surgery training.[25] Additionally, her continued work in data sciences and machine learning has shed new light on the future of surgery. She suggests that surgical data science (SDS) "improves the quality of interventional health care through the capture, organization, analysis, and modeling of data." Her team has been applying these methods in academic surgery and creating roadmaps for faster clinical application of this data. They use AI to assess hours of video capturing surgeons—both masters and novices—to identify differences in techniques, outcomes, and skills. Surgeons' hands were tracked using sensors or markers to understand motion economy and tissue handling.[26] These concepts can easily be applied in OMS with the same sensors and videos capturing common procedures that we conduct. AI can then identify best practices and efficient maneuvers that can translate to teaching and training methodology.

Interpretation of imaging remains an easy task for AI algorithms. OMSs and our trainees interpret thousands of images in our careers without the help of a radiologist. Workflow applications can easily replace the need for a surgeon or trainee spending time reviewing radiographs and then reporting the same in a patient's record. With AI, the OMS would simply be correlating clinical findings and checking for inaccuracies in the interpretation that the algorithm has already presented. There is a lot of focus on developing AI methodology applications in this field to ensure standardized and accurate reporting.[27]

SUMMARY

Artificial intelligence is permeating every aspect of our daily living including the teaching and practice of OMS. Machines that have superior capabilities of speech, natural language, and image recognition are creating neural networks like human synapses and can replicate some of our cognitive capabilities. In theory, these machines can process much more data, much more accurately than humans. Algorithms have the ability to predict patterns of behavior based on what it has learned. Machines are likely to be capable of learning more than humans especially when it comes to multi-dimensional data and predictive patterns. Once it learns patterns, it can make objective predictions and create models that humans cannot even come close to. These qualities of AI are being leveraged in education and medicine and consequently medical education. OMS is uniquely positioned because of the nature of our specialty to be an easy early adopter of AI both in practice and training. The AI awakening is going to be quick and ubiquitous in our specialty.

DISCLOSURE

The authors have nothing to disclose.

REFERENCES

1. Global sensors in internet of Things (IoT) devices market, analysis & Forecast: 2016 to 2022; (focus on Pressure, Temperature, light, Chemical, & motion sensors; and applications in healthcare, Manufacturing, Retail & Transportation). Available at: https://www.researchandmarkets.com/reports/4084655/global-sensors-in-internet-of-things-iot. Accessed November 21 2021.
2. Available at: https://www.researchandmarkets.com/reports/4613290/artificial-intelligence-market-in-the-us Accessed November 21 2021
3. Pinto Dos Santos D, Giese D, Brodehl S, et al. Medical students' attitude towards artificial intelligence: a multicentre survey. Eur Radiol 2019;29(4):1640–6.
4. Gong B, Nugent JP, Guest W, et al. Influence of Artificial Intelligence on Canadian Medical Students' Preference for Radiology Specialty: A National Survey Study. Acad Radiol 2019;26(4):566–77.
5. Blease C, Kharko A, Bernstein M, et al. Machine learning in medical education: a survey of the experiences and opinions of medical students in Ireland. BMJ Health Care Inform 2022;29(1):e100480. https://doi.org/10.1136/bmjhci-2021-100480.
6. Available at: https://www.fda.gov/medical-devices/software-medical-device-samd/artificial-intelligence-and-machine-learning-software-medical-device. Accessed November 21 2021.
7. Available at: https://www.fda.gov/medical-devices/software-medical-device-samd/good-machine-learning-practice-medical-device-development-guiding-principles. Accessed November 22 2021.
8. Lillehaug SI, Lajoie SP. AI in medical education–another grand challenge for medical informatics. Artif Intell Med 1998;12(3):197–225.
9. Sinclair P, Kable A, Levett-Jones T. The effectiveness of internet-based e-learning on clinician behavior and patient outcomes: a systematic review protocol. JBI Database Syst Rev Implement Rep 2015;13(1):52–64. https://doi.org/10.11124/jbisrir-2015-1919.
10. Owolabi J. ASIC Framework Simplified and Operationalised - An Operational Matrix for Optimising the Use of Technologies and Innovations in Medical Education. Adv Med Educ Pract 2022;13:149–56.
11. Grunhut J, Wyatt AT, Marques O. Educating Future Physicians in Artificial Intelligence (AI): An Integrative Review and Proposed Changes. J Med Educ Curric Dev 2021;8. 23821205211036836.
12. Imran N, Jawaid M. Artificial intelligence in medical education: Are we ready for it? Pak J Med Sci 2020;36(5):857–9.
13. Carin, Lawrence PhD. On artificial intelligence and deep learning within medical education, 95 -. Academic Medicine; 2020. p. S10–1. https://doi.org/10.1097/ACM.0000000000003630, 11S.
14. Pereira KR, Sinha R. Welcome the "new kid on the block" into the family: artificial intelligence in oral and maxillofacial surgery. Br J Oral Maxillofac Surg 2020;58(1):83–4.
15. Rekawek P, Rajapakse CS, Panchal N. Artificial Intelligence: The Future of Maxillofacial Prognosis and Diagnosis? J Oral Maxillofac Surg 2021;79(7):1396–7.
16. Mehandru N, Hicks WL Jr, Singh AK, et al. Machine Learning for Identification of Craniomaxillofacial Radiographic Lesions. J Oral Maxillofac Surg 2020;78(12):2106–7.
17. Bas B, Ozgonenel O, Ozden B, et al. Use of artificial neural network in differentiation of subgroups of temporomandibular internal derangements: a preliminary study. J Oral Maxillofac Surg 2012;70(1):51–9.
18. Farook TH, Jamayet NB, Abdullah JY, et al. Machine Learning and Intelligent Diagnostics in Dental and Orofacial Pain Management: A Systematic Review. Pain Res Manag 2021;6659133. https://doi.org/10.1155/2021/6659133.
19. Alabi RO, Youssef O, Pirinen M, et al. Machine learning in oral squamous cell carcinoma: Current status, clinical concerns and prospects for future-A systematic review. Artif Intell Med 2021;115:102060.
20. Karadaghy OA, Shew M, New J, et al. Development and Assessment of a Machine Learning Model to Help Predict Survival Among Patients With Oral Squamous Cell Carcinoma. JAMA Otolaryngol Head Neck Surg 2019;145(12):1115–20.
21. Bur AM, Holcomb A, Goodwin S, et al. Machine learning to predict occult nodal metastasis in early oral squamous cell carcinoma. Oral Oncol 2019;92:20–5.
22. Ding M, Kang Y, Yuan Z, et al. Detection of facial landmarks by a convolutional neural network in patients with oral and maxillofacial disease. Int J Oral Maxillofac Surg 2021;50(11):1443–9.
23. Kesterke MJ, Sankaranarayanan G, Sautter M, et al. March). Saving face: the role of artificial intelligence in evaluating craniofacial variation for the treatment

of orofacial dysfunction. Am J Phys Anthropol 2019; 168:123–4, 111 RIVER ST, HOBOKEN 07030-5774, NJ USA: WILEY.

24. Schwendicke F, Samek W, Krois J. Artificial Intelligence in Dentistry: Chances and Challenges. J Dent Res 2020;99(7):769–74.

25. Korndorffer JR Jr, Hawn MT, Spain DA, et al. Situating Artificial Intelligence in Surgery: A Focus on Disease Severity. Ann Surg 2020;272(3):523–8.

26. Azari DP, Frasier LL, Quamme SRP, et al. Modeling Surgical Technical Skill Using Expert Assessment for Automated Computer Rating. Ann Surg 2019; 269(3):574–81.

27. Putra RH, Doi C, Yoda N, et al. Current applications and development of artificial intelligence for digital dental radiography. Dentomaxillofac Radiol 2022; 51(1):20210197. https://doi.org/10.1259/dmfr. 20210197.

The Aging Surgeon Cohort
Their Impact on the Future of the Specialty

Stephanie J. Drew, DMD[a],*, Leslie R. Halpern, DDS, MD, PHD, MPH, FICD[b]

KEYWORDS

- Aging surgeon • Retirement • Neurocognitive decline • Aging academic surgeon • Generativity

KEY POINTS

- The graying of the surgical workforce will have a profound effect on the quality and access to care, as well as the public safety of the patient population.
- A surgeon should not be mandated to retire at a predetermined age but be objectively assessed and monitored at the appropriate level of competency of his or her surgical skill set throughout his or her career.
- A formal plan to transition from clinical to nonclinical roles should be developed as part of milestones of an academic surgeon's career.
- Longitudinal studies are required to craft accurate and reproducible screening tests that will identify surgeons who are experiencing age-related decline in neurocognitive/surgical skills.
- An academic surgeon emeritus peer group can provide an innovative strategy for career satisfaction of the aging practitioner.

INTRODUCTION

The World Health Organization (WHO) has calculated that the global population is increasing at an annual rate of 1.7%.[1] Those who are aged 65 years or older are increasing at a rate of 2.5%.[1] By 2050, 1 out of 5 persons will be aged 65 years or older. The surgical practitioner is also aging, and this graying of the surgical workforce will influence not only the quality of care being served to the community at hand, but also the physical and mental wellbeing of the practicing physician.[2] It has been said that "excellence in surgery can happen at any age, but the aging surgeon's decades of experience is unparalleled and cannot be taught."[3–5] Greater clinical experience may both benefit patient care, and yet paradoxically, result in poor outcomes depending on the type of procedures performed.[5] Older surgeons in practice perform more poorly on recertification examinations and are less likely to incorporate newer treatment strategies used by their younger cohorts.[5] Other studies, however, support better clinical outcomes of older surgeons than their younger counterparts with respect to operative and postoperative complication rates.[3,5]

With the accumulated life and professional experience obtained, the aging surgeon contributes a valuable perspective/point of view on his or her life and career. Age-related changes in the surgeon, however, can have wider implications when compared with other specialties of medicine and surgery. Many in active clinical practice fear the next phase in their lifespan, specifically, retirement. When should surgeons retire from clinical practice? Many cannot wait to retire, while others continue to be productive regardless of chronologic age because of fear of loss of identity, livelihood, and their status in the community. Decisions to retire are often compounded by a paucity of formal age-based guidelines within their respective specialties.[3,5,6] The American College

[a] Department of Surgery, Division of Oral and Maxillofacial Surgery, Emory University, Atlanta, GA, USA;
[b] Oral and Maxillofacial Surgery, University of Utah School of Dentistry, Salt, Lake City, UT, USA
* Corresponding author.
E-mail address: stephanie.drew@emory.edu

Oral Maxillofacial Surg Clin N Am 34 (2022) 593–601
https://doi.org/10.1016/j.coms.2022.02.005
1042-3699/22/© 2022 Elsevier Inc. All rights reserved.

oralmaxsurgery.theclinics.com

of Surgeons (ACS) measured the average age of surgeons to be greater than 55, and the American Medical Association (AMA) noted that 1 in 4 physicians are greater than age 65.[3] One defense against implementing a mandatory retirement age for surgeons rests in the ability to conduct one's practice based on functional age and not strictly chronologic age.[6]

Many surgeons have chosen an academic career path. Being an academician requires the recognition of the continuum of career growth and the constant evolution of the person teaching. This ideology is most often referred to as generativity, which exemplifies "the propensity and willingness to engage in acts that promote the wellbeing of younger generations as a way of ensuring the long-term survival."[4–6] Senior surgeons possess perspective, history, and skill. When is an academic surgical career over? Or is it? Oral and maxillofacial surgeons (OMFS) who have been in practice for over 3 decades have a great deal of knowledge and wisdom to share. These mentors are now leading the path to the future by training the next generation of surgeon and academicians. The specialty depends on the skillset of an academician to train the future legacy that will fill the voids of surgeons who no longer can provide clinical care. In the absence of a defined retirement age, the academic surgeon can have opportunities for late-career transitioning. The authors present a review article that discusses the current literature on the aging surgeon with respect to the epidemiology of retirement and the neurophysiological, cognitive, and anatomic changes that occur during a surgeon's career; they also suggest strategies for how the aging surgeon can use his or her expertise as an academician in an innovative fashion to train the future legacy of the specialty.

LITERATURE SEARCH

A literature search was undertaken using Medline within the Pub Med portal to choose articles within the last 20 years. Only articles in English were chosen for inclusion. Each article's bibliography was evaluated for relevant publications and reviewed by the authors for inclusion. The keywords chosen included "aging surgeon," "surgical education," "surgery mentor," "generativity," "academic aging," "retirement of surgeons," "oral surgery and retirement," "physician retirement in medicine," and "late-career transitioning for physicians." Other articles were extracted from commentaries across the subspecialties of surgery. The level of evidence chosen was based upon Sacket's hierarchy of evidence.[7] Additional references were

chosen across health disciplines to maintain similarities in terminology that can support this discussion across a wider context.

AGING SURGEONS AND MANDATED RETIREMENT TIMELINES

In the United States, several professions have crafted specific retirement criteria for their workforce where public health safety is at risk.[4,7] Examples include airline pilots, with a mandatory age between 60 and 65, the Federal Bureau of Investigation with mandated retirement at age 57, park rangers at age 57, and air traffic controllers at age 56.[4,7] Globally, the statutory retirement age for a surgeon can vary as policies for surgeon retirement time fluctuate based upon serving in the public and private sectors (**Box 1**).[5,6] In Australia, for example, surgeons are still active at 65. The United Kingdom and Germany have recently phased out mandatory retirement of surgeons in the private sector.[5,6] Within the United States, the Federal Age Discrimination and Employment Act (ADEA) prohibits discrimination on the basis of age for employment of all medical practitioners and surgeons. There are more than 20,000 actively practicing surgeons who are older than age 70.[8] Hummer, in a review article entitled *The Aging Surgeon,* states that there is no age-based definition of physical competence that exists in the United States, and from a surgeon's perspective, retiring from the practice of surgery is considered a negative life transition because of the loss of being a surgeon.[4,9] The variable timeline of a surgeon's career supports a premise that implementing a mandatory retirement age would be unfair. The effects of the aging process

Box 1 Retirement ages for doctors across the globe	
United States of America	No mandatory age
Canada	Minimum age, 65
United Kingdom	No mandatory age
Ireland	Minimum age, 65
Germany	No mandatory age
Italy	No mandatory age
Australia	No mandatory age
India	65 years, public sector only
Russia/China	60 years for men, 55 years for women

Adapted from Bhatt NR, Morris M, O'Neil A, Gillis A, Ridgway PF. When should surgeons retire? Br J Surg. 2016 Jan;103(1):35-42.

can fluctuate among individuals and, as such, functional age may be a more valid measure than chronologic age. The latter requires objective risk predictive tools that have a value for evaluation on competency and care of patients.

HUMAN PHYSIOLOGIC CHANGES AND THE IMPACT ON THE AGING SURGEON

Physiologic and anatomic changes occur during aging that impede a surgeon's skillset. Neuroanatomic changes include shrinkage of the frontal lobes that can impair vision and judgment; increase in size of the ventricles; a reduction in neuron size, quantity, and synapse capabilities; and a decrease in overall healthy brain tissue.[3,5] The motor cortex decreases in ability to reorganize and accommodate new information, and movements become less integrated with cognitive thinking, resulting in a slowing of spatial motor tasks.[3,10–12] The latter causes a decrease in hand dexterity, and a slowing of physical activity, both of which have the potential to impact clinical care (Box 2).

A decline in neurocognitive function with age is characterized by a diminished capacity for focusing attention, correlating information, and speed of processing. Decreased short-term memory and ability to solve problems, and increased reaction time are all risk predictors for surgical error.[2,3,10,11,13] Several studies examined age-related cognitive capacity when physicians are compared with nonphysicians. Although physicians score higher than their nonphysician cohorts, the scores decrease with age in both groups across numerous domains of cognitive function.[3,9] Some neurocognitive functions are preserved, however, such as verbal skills, semantic memory (knowledge of facts and meanings), as well as cumulative knowledge, which exemplifies clinical wisdom referred to as crystallized intelligence.[2,3,14] Evidence supports the aging surgeon to be more adept at nonanalytic diagnostic strategies and pattern recognition.[2,14]

AGE, SURGICAL PERFORMANCE, AND COGNITIVE SKILL STUDIES
Age Criteria

The aging surgeon exemplifies greater experience and wisdom. A paradox, however, finds the opposite to be true. Assuring the competency of surgeons whether they are in middle or late career requires a well calibrated system that can standardize competency with respect to cognitive skills, manual dexterity, and patient care. The responsible agencies to monitor these risk predictors are most often the state, as well as the subspecialty boards of surgery and medicine. Regulations to monitor these predictors, however, are scarce, since a policing within a surgical specialty may fall upon peers that have no rheostat for scrutiny.[2,15] Many state boards can provide process/procedures for disciplinary events but cannot accurately measure the gradual decline in surgical performance and individual error as a surgeon ages.

Surgical Performance

The impact of aging on surgical performance has been objectively scrutinized by data comparing morbidity and mortality of patients treated. Choudry and colleagues in a systematic review found that physicians who have been in practice longer are at risk for providing poorer outcomes in a patient's quality of care.[2,16] Duclos and colleagues suggested that when older surgeons are compared with their younger cohorts, 20 years or more of surgical experience was associated with an increased risk of postoperative complications.[17] Waljee and colleagues provided data suggesting that surgeons aged 60 and over had higher mortality rates than surgeons aged 41 to 50 for procedures (eg, carotid endarterectomy, coronary artery bypass, and pancreatectomy).[3,18] The authors also concluded that there exists an inverse relation between years of surgical experience and knowledge base. Salem-Scharz and colleagues found a significant association between knowledge deficit and the number of years in practice.[2,19,20] Other studies by Tsugawa and colleagues found adjusted operative mortality rates of 6.6%. 6.4%, and 6.3% for surgeons aged under 40 to 49, 50 to 59, and 60 and over, respectively

---

Box 2
Characteristics of the brain and its function with age

Cognitive decline

Deterioration of short-term memory

Decreased reasoning

Adverse effects on attention to details

Regression of higher functions

Reduction in number of synapses

Reduction in volume of brain

Reduced coordination

Manual dexterity is reduced

Sensory impairment: hardening of lens of eye/yellowing/decreased depth perception

(P<.001).[21] The notion that not every surgeon ages the same with respect to knowledge base and experience was measured by Eva, who noted that "variability across the scores individuals receive tends to increase with age and strong individual differences exist."[5]

A paucity of studies exists to correlate surgical performance of older surgeons when compared with younger colleagues using contemporary minimally invasive technology. A study by Powers and colleagues evaluated comfort using minimally invasive laparoscopic instrumentation and concluded that "seasoned surgeons; age greater than 55" had difficulty with minimally invasive instrumentation and relegated its use to their younger colleagues.[22] Many procedures in oral and maxillofacial surgery have been modified or changed over the last 30 years. There have been changes and improvements to trauma management and orthognathic surgery with intermaxillary fixation to plate fixation, dental implant placement, virtual surgical planning in almost all surgery, arthroscopy, robotic surgery, guided surgery, and changing anesthesia techniques. Senior academic surgeons must also learn them, embrace them, and incorporate them in to academic teaching. Who is to say that the experienced academic surgeon could not learn or even create and validate these new ways? Aging academic surgeons should be encouraged to continue to be involved and contribute to the development of the modern standards of care.

Cognitive Skills Studies for Competency

The American College of Surgeons (ACS) crafted a consensus statement on the aging surgeon.[23] Objective assessment by peer-reviewed methods as part of surgeon competency are advised in the recredentialing process. Variables to be measured include practice evaluation, chart reviews, peer review of decision making, patient feedback, and video review of operating room procedures with mentoring of younger surgeons. A comprehensive program should, in addition, be crafted to perform a robust neuropsychological assessment. The ACS further recommends surgeons aged 65 to 70 to undergo voluntary physical examination and visual testing. The costs incurred for testing should fall within the auspices of the hospital center and form part of the overall yearly evaluation of the surgeon including strict confidentiality, respect for the surgeon, and patient safety.

Decisions as to a surgeon's competence with age using these risk predictors, however, can be a daunting task for physician leadership because of the subjective opinions of staff, peers, and trainees. Denial of privileges without objective information can result in acrimony, as well as employment discrimination due to age.[4,23] Currently, there are no standard measurements of neurocognitive and physical testing of older surgeons that can exemplify competency to remain in practice.[2,23,24] Few studies have measured cognitive functions of older surgeons to elucidate the effect of aging on clinical performance.[4,5,24,25] Trunkey and Botnet developed a schema that uses physical examination and a measurement of neurocognitive function using the MicroCog test developed by Powell based on changes in cognitive function, physiology, and psychometrics (**Table 1**).[24,25] Reaction time, numerical recall, verbal memory, visual spatial facility, and mental calculation all declined with age. These results are in line with the standards used by the FAA in recertification of pilots.[24] The authors conclude that aging surgeons should follow the standards of the FAA by undergoing medical evaluation, MicroCog testing, random breathalyzer testing, urine screening and frequency of recertification annually after age 60.[4,24]

Berliauskas and colleagues studied age, cognition and retirement in a group of senior surgeons using the acronym CCRASS (cognitive changes and retirement among senior surgeons). They identified a series of parameters of cognitive aging and their relationship to a surgeon's decision to retire.[26] A computerized battery of cognitive skill tasks focused on visual learning, attention, and reaction time. In addition, a self-report survey was designed to ask the participants their practice status and plans for retirement. The test was administered 5 consecutive years at the ACS annual meeting. The age range tested was 45 years and over, with a total of 359 volunteers (330 men and 29 women, mean age 61.4 years) of whom 294 completed the survey. The authors concluded a need for development of measures of functional aging that will correlate with decisions about retirement and if it is in the best interest of the surgeons and patients they serve.[4,26] The authors also concluded that older surgeons adapt to the decline in cognition by taking more time with their patients, working with others, and seeking second opinions.[2,26] In contrast, Drag and colleagues reviewed the CCRASS study and concluded that most senior surgeons in practice performed almost equal to their younger peers on all cognitive tasks, and as such support the premise that "old age does not inevitably preclude cognitive proficiency."[27]

Another more surgeon-specific solution is the Aging Surgeon Program at the Sinai Hospital of Baltimore. The program is a 2-day process that

Table 1
Contemporary methods in determining surgical competency

Method	Assessment	Validity (PS)	Validity(ST)
MicroCog	5 domains: attention/mental control Memory/calculation/reasoning/spatial/reasoning	Yes	N/A
O-SCORE	Surgical procedure: peer evaluated with a rating Scale: 9 item tools to assess competence to perform A procedure independently	No	Yes
CCRASS	Cognitive changes and retirement among senior Surgeons: visual learning, attention and reaction Time, self-report of desire to retire	Equivocal	N/A
Sinai Hospital Program, MD	Two-day program: objective evaluation of cognition And physical function: confidential report from a Multidisciplinary panel: the program balances patient safety with hospital liability risk while maintaining the dignity of the surgeon	Yes	N/A

Abbreviations: N/A, not applicable multidisciplinary panel; ST, surgical trainee.
  Data from Sataloff RT, Hawkshaw M, Kutinsky J, Maitz EA. The Aging Physician and Surgeon. Ear, Nose & Throat Journal. 2016;95(4-5):1-17.

involves neurologic, neuropsychological, ophthalmologic, and general examination by a third party. At the conclusion of this process and the Stanford screening process, an assessment is made, but there is no specific recommendation on whether the individual should continue to practice (see **Table 1**). Choices of transitioning out of clinical practice may have the potential for increased involvement in more cerebral activities such as mentoring, training students and residents, and research. Future studies are needed with longitudinal testing to establish each surgeon's baseline of cognitive change over time so that consecutive testing scores during the later years can be interpreted more meaningfully. The latter is essential in order to correlate these results with surgeon privileges at their respective institutions.[4,28]

THE FUTURE OF ACADEMIA AND THE AGING SURGEON
Innovative Technology

The first year of COVID-19 challenged all of academia to rethink teaching. Faculty members had to learn and adopt new methods of teaching and sharing of information across learning platforms not previously explored . Computer technology had already become an essential tool in the academic armamentarium in a single health center. The pandemic has afforded an opportunity for innovative collaboration among academic institutions. The sharing of knowledge in areas of expertise via an online platform has given

residents access to several paradigms within the OMS arena not available at their own home base. This opportunity has opened up new ways for how collaboration will continue across the specialty. The sense of academic community has never been stronger.

The future of academia will also begin to rely upon virtual reality and artificial intelligence to be incorporated into new learning platforms to test for competency of trainees and senior surgeons in a fair and quantitative way. There are already many tests for cognitive function used today in medicine and surgery. The age of the surgeon will not matter, just skill and competence. Surgical competency may be measured by developing technology to test for hand-eye coordination, decision making, and reaction times specific to a specialty. Valid, reliable, and feasible ways of testing surgical skill competence have been introduced to the otolaryngology training programs on a procedural basis.[29] They used a task specific checklist with a global rating scale. They also documented their feedback and a final decision as to the ability of achieving autonomy by the resident trainee for the procedure. These programs can help institutions become safer spaces for patients, residents, and attending surgeons. Other computer programs will need to be developed by senior and young academic surgeons collaborating with computer engineers. These new tools will allow one to check for competency and then immediately provide feedback for remediate in a safe environment. In addition, not only will these tools be used for residents, but for experienced surgeons who perhaps want to rehearse a patient-specific procedure and practice if they have not done a specific procedure for a long time. The ultimate goal is to train the future generation so surgeons can become both independent and trustworthy in the care of patients.

Experience leads to knowledge, and then knowledge leads to wisdom. A more experienced academic surgeon provides a source of expertise that comes with the ability to guide unskilled hands with confidence in the clinic and the operating room. While the future of learning may use virtual platforms and artificial intelligence to assess learning, as the resident proceeds through training, the assessments will be done in the operating room by experienced hands. There will always be a place at the table for competent surgeons who can teach in the clinical setting. Senior surgeons can call upon their knowledge and experience and wisdom when unexpected events happen while operating (ie, teaching younger surgeons how to problem solve in real time).

Humanities in Surgery and the Aging Academic Surgeon

With the accumulated life and professional experience obtained, the aging surgeon can contribute a valuable perspective/point of view by teaching how the principles of humanities form a strong foundation in surgical practice . Teaching ethics, cultural competence, medical-legal issues, professionalism, negotiation and business, leadership, citizenship, and critical thinking are just a small list of what can be delivered by an experienced surgeon. Academic institutions must consider the value of these faculty members, The aging surgeon can provide a segue by introducing trainees to critical thinking, analytical reasoning, health activism, the history of surgery, effects of gender and disability variables—topics that may be unfamiliar but encompass issues that all should grapple with, including how bias, race-based medicine, and societal structures have hindered a level playing field for better health outcomes for all ethnicities, gender, and races.

Museum-based education teaches critical thinking skills (SJD, personal communication).[30] The museum is also a powerful resource for anatomic studies, using sculptures and drawing techniques taught not only to improve hand to eye coordination but also as a tool to communicate. Visual thinking strategies are used to develop deep observation, reflection, and discussion. One of the authors, SJD, is involved in a multidisciplinary group of doctors bringing humanities and medical/surgical education to the forefront with museum-based education utilization as a tool to teach dexterity, observational skills, communication skills and empathy. This promotes awareness of biases, metacognition, tolerance of uncertainty, enhanced observation skills, broadening of differential diagnosis, joy in practice, and flattening of the perceived medical hierarchy.[31] The comradery of well-seasoned surgeons from all health specialties has the potential for increased creativity, satisfaction and purpose in this period of their lives .

The Academic Oral and Maxillofacial Surgeon Emeritus

Judith Hall, professor emerita states, "It seems a waste of human capital not to utilize the hard-won skills of academia during our later years in new and creative ways.......older academics make new types of contributions to society."[32] The surgeon emeritus concept can be an innovative strategy for creating the next and final phase in an OMFS surgeon's career. While trading a scalpel for a pencil or paint brush seems like a compromise, it is essential for the development of the future generation of academic surgeons. Experience, wisdom, and mentoring are essential for success. Clinical retirement does not mean surgeons are not able to be productive or successful as academicians. Surgeons by nature typically look for mental stimulation and physical activity. In order to do this, one must remain healthy physically and mentally. One must be financially sound, have hobbies and family and friends, and something to do each day that makes one feel valid; the surgeon also must always seek to grow and learn. Continuing to serve one's institution in some way may provide this daily validation (**Box 3**). For instance, intellectual stimulation comes with the act of preparing didactic lessons and teaching. This simple act allows the senior surgeon a way to contribute to the specialty and give back. Topics such as surgical anatomy, history and evolution of surgical procedures, physical examination skills, and basic surgical skills would be well taught by the surgeon emeritus. These types of lesson plans would serve medical school, dental school, and residency education well.

Volunteering as a senior surgeon on mission trips may be a rewarding experience for those who did not have the opportunity to do so during their career. Imagine the emeritus as a group leader coordinating the mission trip, assessing patients, and preparing them for surgery. Continuity of patient care is often difficult because of the time restrictions of volunteer surgeons; a senior

---

Box 3
Innovative strategies where the surgeon emeritus can make an impact

- Develop validation studies on competence testing
- Participate in the development of current standards of care for OMS
- Incorporate humanities into medical/surgical education
- Volunteer on mission trips as a coordinator and mission specialist
- Serve on institutional committees as a consultant
- Serve the institution by teaching and improving the didactic curriculum
- Remain active in research.
- Mentor
- Develop courses to groom the next generation of academicians
- Develop and implement the academic emeritus peer group

---

programming and training of the next generation of surgeons. Too many have not planned and left the helm to the inexperienced academic, where grit and resilience were needed to upright that ship and keep it sailing. It would be far better to be prepared and to leave a sustainable program and legacy of which they are proud.

Although each institution may have leadership courses available, there is also a need for the AAOMS, ACOMS, and the ACS to develop courses related to the specifics of OMS education academics and academic leaders. There have been many business leadership courses available, but no consistent ones in academic leadership, that should be required for all OMS academia to attend throughout their careers. Topics such as career development, research and collaboration among programs (we are stronger together), managing a department, leading a team, understanding strategic planning, and managing a budget are a few categories that the emeriti could help develop. These courses should be created and led by academic OMS emeriti.

WHAT IS NEXT: THE RESPONSIBILITIES OF BUILDING AN ACADEMIC OMS EMERITUS COLLEGE PEER GROUP AND COMMUNITY BUILDING

The human capital of age is wisdom. Collaboration of the academic OMS emeritus force is a must. Serving on committees and councils to provide perspective and share knowledge and advice should be strongly recommended by department chairs. Advisory boards to AAOMS, ACOMS, and ACS academic and nonacademic communities would be remiss in their duties without a variety of generations and genders serving. Mentoring and coaching will be needed for the development future academic leaders. It will be necessary to have a pool of able emeriti to volunteer and step up to ensure the specialty remains strong.

The OMS emeritus group shares the responsibility of contributing to teaching how to avoid disasters from the masters' to prevent future failures. These pearls of wisdom are essential to give back to the next generation in order for the specialty to grow. The emeritus surgeon will be able to continue to contribute a great deal to the specialty. The authors recognize the fact that age-related changes may contribute to an inability to continue with clinical practice. Realistically, age-related cognitive and skills testing should be implemented as a way to protect the public, the institution, and the surgeon. The OMS emeritus group should be involved in developing this testing. The favor of mandatory testing of physical

surgeon emeritus can potentially remain in place longer at a site to assist the local teams during the postoperative periods. They can also be in command of teaching the local doctors and health care providers to make the patient care sustainable once the team leaves.

Remaining active in research activities will also be important as a contribution to the specialty. Writing grants, coming up with research proposals, leading a research team, and compiling important data are a few ways to remain involved. The emeritus as an inventor can also use experience and wisdom to improve the way things are done. Imaging improving on surgical instrumentation, procedure modifications or developing new methods to improve outcomes and patient safety? How many times has a surgeon been in the operating room and wished he or she had an instrument that did "this"?

THE ACADEMIC SURGEON EMERITUS ROLE AS A PRODUCER OF NEW ACADEMIC LEADERS

The next generation of academic leaders needs to be carefully cultivated by the senior professors. Preparing for emeritus status comes with the responsibility to plan for the future and develop the next person in line to take the helm. This type of coaching, mentoring, and leadership development is essential to the survival of academic dexterity, cognitive skills, and hand/eye coordination should be tested starting at the age of 65 and at least every 2 years. Licensing agencies should delegate authority to test fellow doctors to the peer review organizations and work with surgical associations to ensure that surgeons' rights and due process are upheld.

As described previously, there are institutions that have testing available. The Aging Surgeon Program sponsored by Sinai Hospital of Baltimore and Life Bridge Health, and the Physician Assessment and Clinical Education Program (PACE) at the University of California San Diego provide these services. They are centers that are available to doctors around the country and not specific to OMS. They provide assessment of impairment related to substance abuse, other mental health disorders, and medical illness.[31,33] Members of this specialty must be proactive instead of reactive with developing this assessment. It is best left to each surgical specialty to set its own standards. The OMS emeritus group would make great contributions in setting up these benchmarks. The next step would be to establish a task force to identify and validate these methods of functional age and cognitive testing related to surgeons and ultimately, provide a value regarding protecting both the surgeon and the public.

As surgeons each enter into the sunset of their careers, they cannot help but believe that there is so much work to be done on this front to prepare for the future generations of academicians. The authors look forward to developing the next generation of academic emeriti and surgeons to secure the future as a specialty. The authors also look forward to continuing to contribute in meaningful ways to patients, residents, and the specialty.

DISCLOSURE

The authors do not have any relationship with a commercial company that has a direct financial interest in subject matter or materials discussed in the article or with a company making a competing product.

REFERENCES

1. Razak PA, Richard KMJ, Thankachan RP, et al. Geriatric oral health: a review article. J Int Oral Health 2014;6(6):110–6.
2. Schenarts PJ, Cernaj S. The aging surgeon: implications for the workforce, the surgeon, and the patient. Surg Clin NA 2016;96:126–38.
3. Asserson DB, Janis JE. The aging surgeon: evidence and experience. Aesthet Surg J 2021;1–7.
4. Sataloff RT, Hawkshaw M, Kutinsky J, et al. The aging physician and surgeon. Ear, Nose Throat J 2020; 95(4–5):E35–47.
5. Bhatt NR, Morris M, O'Neil A, et al. When should surgeons retire? Br J surg 2015;103:35–43.
6. Richards R, Mcleod R, Latter D, et al. Toward late career transitioning: a proposal for academic surgeons. Can J Surg 2017;60(5):355–8.
7. Sadoski SJ, Fitzpatrick B, Curtis DA. Evidence-based criteria for different treatment planning of implant restorations for the maxillary edentulous patient. J Prosth 2015;433–46.
8. Katlic MA, Coleman J. The aging surgeon. Adv Surg 2016;50:93–103.
9. Hummer CD. The aging surgeon: how old is too old? AAOS Now. 2007. Available at. http://www.aaos.org/news/bulletin/may07/managing4.asp. Accessed December 13, 2021.
10. Gallagher AG, Satava RM, O'Sullivan GC. Attention al capacity: an essential aspect of surgical performance. Ann Surg 2015;261(3):e60–1.
11. Hickson GB, Peabody T, Hopkinson WJ, et al. Cognitive skills assessment for the aging orthopedic surgeon: AOA critical issues. J Bone Joint Surg Am 2019;101(2):e7.
12. Voelcker-Rehage C, Alberts JL. Age-related changes in grasping force modulation. Exp Brain Res 2005;166(1):61–70.
13. Powell DH, Whittle DK. Profiles in cognitive aging. Cambridge, MA: Harvard University Press; 1994.
14. Turnbull J, Cunnington J, Unsal A, et al. Competence and cognitive difficulty in physicians : a follow-up study. Acad Med 2006;81:915–9.
15. Burroughs J. Dealing with the aging physician: advocacy or betrayal? Physician Exec 2012;38(6):38–41.
16. Choudry NK, Fletcher RH, Soumerai SB. Systematic review: the relationship between clinical experience and quality of healthcare. Ann Int Med 2003;142:260–73.
17. Duclos A, Peix JL, Colin C, et al. Influence of experience on performance of individual surgeons in thyroid surgery; prospective cross-sectional multicenter study. Br Med J 2012;344:d8041.
18. Waljee JF, Greenfield LJ, Dimick JB, et al. Surgeon age and operative mortality in the United States. Ann Surg 2006;244(3):353–62.
19. Salem-Schatz SR, Avorn J, Soumerai SB. Influence of clinical knowledge, organizational context and practice style on transfusion decision making: Implications for practice change strategies. JAMA 1990; 264:476–83.
20. Eva KW. The aging physician :changes in cognitive processing and their impact on medical practice. Acad Med 2002;77(Suppl):S1–6.
21. Tsugawa Y, Jena AB, Orav EJ, et al. Age and sex of surgeons and mortality of older surgical patients: observational study. Br Med J 2018;361:k1343.

22. Powers K, Rehrig ST, Schwaizberg SD, et al. Seasoned surgeons assessed in a laparoscopic surgical crisis. J Gastrointest Surg 2009;13:994–1003.

23. American College of Surgeons. Statement on the aging surgeon. Available at: https://www.facs.org/about-acs/statements/80-aging-surgeon. Accessed December 16, 2021.

24. Trunkey DD, Botney R. Assessing competency: a tale of two professions. J Am Coll Surg 2001;192:385–95.

25. Powell DH. Profiles in cognitive aging. Cambridge, MA: Harvard University Press; 1994.

26. Bieliauskas LA, Langenecker SA, Graver C, et al. Cognitive changes and retirement among senior surgeons (CCRASS): Results from the CCEASS study. J Am Coll Surg 2008;207:69–79.

27. Drag LL, Bieliauskas LA, Langenecker SA, et al. Cognitive functioning, retirement status, age: Results from the Cognitive changes and Retirement Among Senior Surgeons study. J Am Coll Surg 2010;211:303–7.

28. Frazer A, Tanzer M. Hangin gup the surgical cap: Assessing the competence of aging surgeons. World J Orthoped 2021;12(4):234–45.

29. Obeid AA, Al-Qahtani KH, Ashraf M, et al. Development and testing for an operative competency assessment tool for nasal septoplasty surgery. Am J Rhinol Allergy 2014;28(4):e163–7.

30. Gooding HC, Quinn M, Martin B, et al. Fostering humanism in medicine through At and reflection. J Mus Education 2016;41:123–30.

31. Naghshineh S, Hafler JP, Miller AR, et al. Formal art observation training improves medical students' visual diagnostic skills. J Gen Intern Med 2008;23:991–7.

32. Hall JG. Continuing contributions of older academics. Am J Med Gen 2021;185A:647–57.

33. Vick DJ. Should Surgeons have a mandatory retirement age? – a number may be arbitrary, but age-related cognitive and skills testing can protect patients. Medpage Today 2021. Available at: www.medpagetoday.com.

Statement of Ownership, Management, and Circulation
UNITED STATES POSTAL SERVICE® (All Periodicals Publications Except Requester Publications)

1. Publication Title	2. Publication Number	3. Filing Date
ORAL & MAXILLOFACIAL SURGERY CLINICS OF NORTH AMERICA	006 – 362	9/18/2022

4. Issue Frequency	5. Number of Issues Published Annually	6. Annual Subscription Price
FEB, MAY, AUG, NOV	4	$405.00

7. Complete Mailing Address of Known Office of Publication (Not printer) (Street, city, county, state, and ZIP+4®)

ELSEVIER INC.
230 Park Avenue, Suite 800
New York, NY 10169

Contact Person
Malathi Samayan

Telephone (Include area code)
91-44-4299-4507

8. Complete Mailing Address of Headquarters or General Business Office of Publisher (Not printer)

ELSEVIER INC.
230 Park Avenue, Suite 800
New York, NY 10169

9. Full Names and Complete Mailing Addresses of Publisher, Editor, and Managing Editor (Do not leave blank)

Publisher (Name and complete mailing address)

Dolores Meloni, ELSEVIER INC.
1600 JOHN F KENNEDY BLVD. SUITE 1800
PHILADELPHIA, PA 19103-2899

Editor (Name and complete mailing address)

JOHN VASSALLO, ELSEVIER INC.
1600 JOHN F KENNEDY BLVD. SUITE 1800
PHILADELPHIA, PA 19103-2899

Managing Editor (Name and complete mailing address)

PATRICK MANLEY, ELSEVIER INC.
1600 JOHN F KENNEDY BLVD. SUITE 1800
PHILADELPHIA, PA 19103-2899

10. Owner (Do not leave blank. If the publication is owned by a corporation, give the name and address of the corporation immediately followed by the names and addresses of all stockholders owning or holding 1 percent or more of the total amount of stock. If not owned by a corporation, give the names and addresses of the individual owners. If owned by a partnership or other unincorporated firm, give its name and address as well as those of each individual owner. If the publication is published by a nonprofit organization, give its name and address.)

Full Name	Complete Mailing Address
WHOLLY OWNED SUBSIDIARY OF REED/ELSEVIER, US HOLDINGS	1600 JOHN F KENNEDY BLVD. SUITE 1800 PHILADELPHIA, PA 19103-2899

11. Known Bondholders, Mortgagees, and Other Security Holders Owning or Holding 1 Percent or More of Total Amount of Bonds, Mortgages, or Other Securities. If none, check box ▶ ☐ None

Full Name	Complete Mailing Address
N/A	

12. Tax Status (For completion by nonprofit organizations authorized to mail at nonprofit rates) (Check one)
The purpose, function, and nonprofit status of this organization and the exempt status for federal income tax purposes:
☒ Has Not Changed During Preceding 12 Months
☐ Has Changed During Preceding 12 Months (Publisher must submit explanation of change with this statement)

PS Form 3526, July 2014 [Page 1 of 4 (see instructions page 4)] PSN: 7530-01-000-9931   PRIVACY NOTICE: See our privacy policy on www.usps.com

---

13. Publication Title	14. Issue Date for Circulation Data Below
ORAL & MAXILLOFACIAL SURGERY CLINICS OF NORTH AMERICA	MAY 2022

15. Extent and Nature of Circulation		Average No. Copies Each Issue During Preceding 12 Months	No. Copies of Single Issue Published Nearest to Filing Date
a. Total Number of Copies (Net press run)		620	546
b. Paid Circulation (By Mail and Outside the Mail)	(1) Mailed Outside-County Paid Subscriptions Stated on PS Form 3541 (Include paid distribution above nominal rate, advertiser's proof copies, and exchange copies)	487	449
	(2) Mailed In-County Paid Subscriptions Stated on PS Form 3541 (Include paid distribution above nominal rate, advertiser's proof copies, and exchange copies)	0	0
	(3) Paid Distribution Outside the Mails Including Sales Through Dealers and Carriers, Street Vendors, Counter Sales, and Other Paid Distribution Outside USPS®	74	57
	(4) Paid Distribution by Other Classes of Mail Through the USPS (e.g., First-Class Mail®)	0	0
c. Total Paid Distribution (Sum of 15b (1), (2), (3), and (4)) ▶		561	506
d. Free or Nominal Rate Distribution (By Mail and Outside the Mail)	(1) Free or Nominal Rate Outside-County Copies included on PS Form 3541	43	25
	(2) Free or Nominal Rate In-County Copies Included on PS Form 3541	0	0
	(3) Free or Nominal Rate Copies Mailed at Other Classes Through the USPS (e.g., First-Class Mail)	0	0
	(4) Free or Nominal Rate Distribution Outside the Mail (Carriers or other means)	0	0
e. Total Free or Nominal Rate Distribution (Sum of 15d (1), (2), (3) and (4)) ▶		43	25
f. Total Distribution (Sum of 15c and 15e) ▶		604	531
g. Copies not Distributed (See instructions to Publishers #4 (page #3)) ▶		16	15
h. Total (Sum of 15f and g) ▶		620	546
i. Percent Paid (15c divided by 15f times 100) ▶		92.88%	95.29%

* If you are claiming electronic copies, go to line 16 on page 3. If you are not claiming electronic copies, skip to line 17 on page 3.

PS Form 3526, July 2014 (Page 2 of 4)

16. Electronic Copy Circulation	Average No. Copies Each Issue During Preceding 12 Months	No. Copies of Single Issue Published Nearest to Filing Date
a. Paid Electronic Copies ▶		
b. Total Paid Print Copies (Line 15c) + Paid Electronic Copies (Line 16a) ▶		
c. Total Print Distribution (Line 15f) + Paid Electronic Copies (Line 16a) ▶		
d. Percent Paid (Both Print & Electronic Copies) (16b divided by 16c × 100) ▶		

☒ I certify that 50% of all my distributed copies (electronic and print) are paid above a nominal price.

17. Publication of Statement of Ownership
☒ If the publication is a general publication, publication of this statement is required. Will be printed in the NOVEMBER 2022 issue of this publication.   ☐ Publication not required.

18. Signature and Title of Editor, Publisher, Business Manager, or Owner

Malathi Samayan   Date 9/18/2022

Malathi Samayan - Distribution Controller

I certify that all information furnished on this form is true and complete. I understand that anyone who furnishes false or misleading information on this form or who omits material or information requested on the form may be subject to criminal sanctions (including fines and imprisonment) and/or civil sanctions (including civil penalties).

PS Form 3526, July 2014 (Page 3 of 4)   PRIVACY NOTICE: See our privacy policy on www.usps.com

Printed and bound by CPI Group (UK) Ltd, Croydon, CR0 4YY

08/05/2025

01864723-0015